Individualised Care: The Role of the Ward Sister

Roswyn A Brown
MPhil, BA, SRN, SCM, DN(Lond), CertEd, RNT

Submitted for the degree of
Master of Philosophy from the
University of Warwick

ROYAL COLLEGE OF NURSING
RESEARCH SERIES

Scutari Press

Aims of the Series

To encourage the appreciation and dissemination of nursing research by making relevant studies of high quality available to the profession at reasonable cost.

The RCN is happy to publish this series of research reports. The projects were chosen by the individual research worker and the findings are those of the researcher and relate to the particular subject in the situation in which it was studied. The RCN in accordance with its policy of promoting research awareness among members of the profession commends this series for study but views expressed do not necessarily reflect RCN policy.

Scutari Press

Viking House, 17–19 Peterborough Road,
Harrow, Middlesex HA1 2AX, England

A subsidiary of Scutari Projects, the publishing company of
the Royal College of Nursing

British Library Cataloguing in Publication Data:

Brown, Roswyn A.
  Individualised care : the role of the ward sister.
  (Royal College of Nursing Research Series ; ISSN (0956–8395)
  1. Great Britain. Hospitals. Wards. Management. Role of Ward sister
  1. Title II. Series
  362.1'1'068

ISBN 1–871364–25–6

Typeset by Action Typesetting Ltd., Gloucester
Printed and bound in Great Britain by Billing & Sons, Worcester

H ⌄ H 7767 /11·50 . 1·92

Contents

Acknowledgements

My first thanks must go to those parents and children who permitted me to share not only their triumphs but also their pain, and to the two ward sisters and their staff, who had the courage to allow me to scrutinise their professional practice.

Thanks are also due to Professor Margaret Stacey and Dr Helen Evers, who so patiently supervised the research on which this book is based. Pat Burford and Judith Edney gave valuable secretarial support. My husband, Alan, and children, Eleanor and Matthew, have not only acquired and contributed considerable information technology skills but have also continued to love me in the process; for this, my gratitude is boundless. Finally, I am grateful to my friends, colleagues and students for the supportive gift relationships that they have so generously shared with me during this time.

Roswyn Brown

For

my father, Hector, and my daughter, Eleanor

'Paradise lost, Paradise regained'

Summary

This study was carried out in two medical wards of a children's hospital. The aim was to examine whether there was any relationship between patterns of work organisation and the provision of individual care. The research focused on the ward sisters' work concepts, how they carried these out and how the sick children experienced their care.

The literature relating to work organisation, the care of sick children in hospital and standards of care is reviewed. Data relating to the ward sisters were obtained by semi-structured interviews and non-participant observation over a 3-day period. Selected children were observed from admission for up to 4 days, using a combination of diary records and time sampling.

The interviews with the ward sisters indicated the way they saw their work, either in terms of patient- or task-centredness. The 3-day observations of the sisters' work tended to confirm what they said in the interviews.

An analysis of the experiences of the children showed that the children on the patient allocation ward received patient-centred care, both during the admission period and subsequently during their hospital stay. Conversely, care tended to be task-centred on the task allocation ward.

It is argued that the style of work organisation is rather less crucial to patient- or task-centred approaches to patient care than was at first believed. Rather, it was how the sisters saw their work and carried it out that was of primary importance in influencing the style of the interactions of the staff with the sick children. It is asserted that the quality of care, using an individualised approach, is closely associated with the quality of social interaction, and that the sister's position is central to this, in terms of the role model that she provides.

Preface

This research originated from a growing personal concern with the care that was being offered to patients by nurses. This concern has spanned a professional nursing career that has lasted nearly 30 years, and which has itself encompassed several significant life events, such as becoming in turn a ward sister, a wife, a nurse tutor, a mother and, last but certainly not least, a patient.

Each new role further reinforced the growing realisation that something very essential was absent from the nursing care I was either giving or receiving. It is likely that the new relationships of wife and mother that I took on threw into sharp relief the different processes of caring that occurred in the two arenas of home and hospital. The contrast appeared to focus on the notion that in hospital sick people took on the 'persona' of the illness state, with the 'self' becoming subjugated to this new emphasis, while at home the reverse appeared to be the norm.

This denial of the patients' identity seemed to me to be the epitome of brutality in its most refined and sophisticated form, particularly when perpetrated under the guise of 'health care'.

Hospitals are, by their very nature, distressing places. I began to wonder exactly what it was that we did to add to that distress, which culminated in the loss of each patient's self-identity.

My thoughts began to centre around methods of work organisation as a possible means of refocusing nursing attention on the patient as an individual. I became particularly interested in two contrasting modes of work organisation, notably task and patient allocation. Well-known nurses and others expounded the suitability of patient allocation as a means of delivering individualised care to the patient. If this was really so, why was it that patient allocation had not really caught on? This was further complicated by the official adoption of the nursing process by the statutory body, a necessary prerequisite of which seemed to be a system of patient allocation. Clearly it was becoming more urgent to examine patient allocation. What did it look like? Did it do the things that people believed it did, e.g. provide a better standard of care that was individualistic by nature? By the same token, it became important to carry out a parallel examination of task allocation. Was task allocation so very bad for patients? If it was, why was it? Could care be individualised using a system of task allocation?

Dickoff et al (1975) rightly point out that '. . . research activity can become occupational therapy to distract the inquirer from the painful practice situation' (p.89). The research design took account of this. The data collection was a painful process. Watching sick children suffer was even more difficult than actually providing their care. In addition, it was distressing to invade the professional privacy of practising nurses. It was always important to try to provide what Fretwell (1980) describes as a 'pay off' for nursing.

Perhaps we should leave June Jolly (1981, p.42) to have the final word:

> 'Nothing can take the place of human contact. Each sick child is an individual and has the right to be treated with respect, which demands that we care enough to listen to what is being said to us. We need to get alongside each young patient and his parents as they struggle with hospital and sickness, but we also need the ability and determination to interpret the truth with love.'

1 The organisation of nursing work

INTRODUCTION

The aim of this research was to describe and analyse the pattern of work organisation used in each of two paediatric wards in the medical unit of a children's hospital. Each ward had its own ward sister, and the unit as a whole was managed by one nursing officer.

The two types of work organisation being investigated were task and patient allocation. The meanings of these terms (and others used synonymously) will be considered more fully later. In particular, it was intended to examine the popular notion (as evidenced by the large numbers of published opinions of practising nurses, e.g. Matthews, 1972; Pembrey, 1975; Plumpton, 1978) that a patient allocation type of work organisation has the potential to confront some of the negative outcomes for sick children in the ward environment. Evidence of negative outcomes is amply provided in the literature (e.g. Stacey et al, 1970; Hawthorn, 1974; Menzies, 1975; Hall, 1977; Jacobs, 1979; Hall and Stacey, 1979), which suggests that hospitalisation is particularly distressing to children, who do not have the social skills necessary to provide the emotional capital to support themselves or others in stressful situations.

The objectives of the study were threefold:

- to identify, compare and contrast patient and task allocation;
- to establish the contribution of the ward sister in relation to the mode of work organisation;
- to compare and contrast patient experiences in two settings using the different modes of work organisation.

1

A PUBLIC IDEOLOGY

As long ago as 1959, the Platt Report said that children in hospital would especially benefit from a system of patient allocation:

> 'For the child's own welfare, a method of nursing which gives him a sense of security through being nursed by a familiar person, as in patient or case assignment, is preferable to other systems.'

It is likely that this stance that was being adopted by Platt was informed by earlier work (Bowlby, 1951; Robertson, 1958) concerning the effects on children of institutionalisation and maternal deprivation.

The notion postulated by Platt (1959) of patient allocation providing a means for improving the quality of the sick child's experience of hospital was echoed by another public report in 1972 (Report of the Committee on Nursing, the Briggs Report). The Briggs Report was concerned mainly with making recommendations for nurse training. However, it did address the problem of work organisation in relation to nurse satisfaction and patient welfare.

Surveys showed that only 31% of nurses sampled favoured task allocation, while 71% regarded patient allocation as best for the comfort of the patient (Briggs Report, 1972, para.124). Despite this, the Report asserted that in acute hospitals '61% of the work is allocated by task' (para.124).

The Briggs Report also suggested that much of the frustration expressed by nursing personnel was due to a production-line concept of care, and that the right approach to care was one that was patient orientated, so that the patient was, at all times, kept as the focus of the activities that were being carried out. The Report stated that, at its worst, task allocation could make the routine more important than the patient (para.122).

These two policy documents represent a public ideology that has expressed, first, a dissatisfaction with the quality of care that children receive in hospital, and, second, a concern with the level of work satisfaction achieved by the nurses in relation to the care they are delivering. It was suggested that the solution to both of these dilemmas could be found in the reorganisation of the work on a patient allocation basis.

THE PROFESSIONAL IDEOLOGY

Platt (1959) was not the first to suggest the use of work reorganisation as a means of delivering improved patient care. The nursing profession itself had drawn attention to this problem in the form of a Royal College of Nursing (RCN) statement on nursing policy (Royal College of Nursing, 1956), which suggested that the resources of the hospital ward should be organised to ensure not only that the physical needs of the patients were met, but also that their sense of confidence and security was built up. To this end, the RCN recommended that care should be delivered using a 'team' approach (see Metcalfe, 1982, p.11).

Since that time, practising nurses have written numerous articles for the nursing press, in which they have related their own personal experiences of patient allocation and have made assertions about the efficacy of this style of work organisation in terms of good standards of care (e.g. Jenkinson, 1958, 1961; Matthews, 1972; Pembrey, 1975).

In an overview of the above literature, the following assumed advantages for the patient have been extracted and summarised as follows:

- less fragmented care;
- the patient's individual needs becoming more apparent;
- an individualised patient-centred, rather than ward-centred, approach;
- an improved nurse–patient relationship;
- an increased feeling of safety and security;
- increased opportunity to rest.

As a result of the practitioners' own experiences, it was believed that task allocation did not achieve the above advantages and that, while there were certain problems that would be encountered in the patient allocation system (notably that it was prone to revert to task allocation unless stable staffing levels were maintained), it was considered to be a much superior and more worthwhile method of organising the delivery of nursing care. The advantages demonstrated not only an increasing awareness of the importance of the patient's psychosocial needs and the individuality of those needs, but also the increasing professionalism of nurses. Metcalfe

(1982, p.2) notes that:

> 'Supporters of this "professionalism" maintain that nurses are not the "handmaidens" of the doctors, but are, or should be, able to accept and exercise considerable responsibility, autonomy and discretion, in their own area of expertise – nursing care.'

Thus, patient allocation had not only become associated with individualised care and 'patient-centredness', but it had also become associated with the professionalisation of nursing and 'nurse-centredness'. Clearly, it is crucial that the profession should be aware of the tension that these dimensions could produce and that there could be a danger that nurse-centredness might be allowed to subsume the interests of patient welfare, if the right balance was not achieved between the two dimensions.

In recent years, more sophisticated members of the profession have been presenting increasingly complex notions of definitions relating to task and patient allocation. A state of some confusion exists relating to what is being defined. Are they all describing the same phenomena? Are the terms directly interchangeable? What do these approaches look like when they are implemented, and what results do they achieve? Are these results different?

Pembrey's (1980) comprehensive statement highlights rather than disentangles this confusion when she says:

> 'The issue of individualised and non-individualised nursing is important enough for nurses to have developed terms to distinguish between individualised and non-individualised nursing. Thus, nursing which recognises the patient as an individual is described as total patient care, patient centred care or patient allocation/while nursing where the patient is not recognised as an individual is termed routine care, job centred nursing or task allocation.'

However, Pembrey does go on to imply that the profession could mean different things in the usage of these particular terms:

> 'a variety of meanings is attached to these words from a symbolic representation (Bendall, 1975) to a means of describing nurse deployment (Kratz, 1974).'

Metcalfe (1982) acknowledges the difficulty that has arisen in the confusion of the nomenclature, compounded perhaps by the advent of the nursing process.

THE NURSING PROCESS AND PROFESSIONALISM

The nursing process began to emerge as a professional ideology in the United States in the 1950s. It consisted of a systematic method for identifying patients' problems, developing plans to resolve them, implementing the plans and evaluating whether they had been effective. By the mid 1970s, it was well on the way to becoming an institution, inasmuch as it became a 'prerequisite for the accreditation of nursing services' (De la Cuesta, 1983, p.367).

De la Cuesta's (1983) excellent overview of the sociological development of the nursing process sought to explain the reasons for the professional adoption of this particular model of care, as a response to 'major structural changes in American society and medicine' (p.367). These changes focused around increased opportunities for higher education, a developing feminist consciousness, expansion of medical and sociological knowledge, the development of auxiliary health occupations, increased health-care costs and an accompanying rise in public expectations. In addition to these societal changes, the nursing profession itself was manifesting feelings of dissatisfaction with its own status and with the quality of care that it was offering to the public.

The North American experience of the 1970s with the nursing process was, to some extent, being paralleled in Britain in terms of patient allocation, since both notions were concerned with ideas of nurse-centredness as well as patient-centredness. It was, therefore, to some extent unsurprising that a natural sequence to this state of affairs should be the wholesale adoption (admittedly in a modified form) of the nursing process in Britain. Metcalfe (1982, p.33) stated that:

> 'The benefits of a system of individualised care for both patients and nursing staff, previously associated with a system of Patient Allocation have been transferred to the "Nursing Process" and a system of Patient Allocation has been relegated to mean no more than the particular method of deploying nurses.'

De la Cuesta (1983) implied that the adoption of the nursing process in Britain had more altruistic origins: 'Nurses were unhappy with the existing system of delivering care and were seeking more satisfactory methods of nursing ...'

She noted the pre-1970s solution to these problems, e.g. patient assignment and total patient care, and traced the progress of the nursing process from initial professional discussions in 1973 to official recognition, in the form of inclusion in the syllabus of statutory training in 1977, and to the publication of the first book on it in 1979. De la Cuesta concluded that:

'The Nursing Process was seen more in terms of a method to improve quality of care and the nurses' satisfaction than a vehicle to achieve professional status . . .' (p.368)

It is beyond the remit of this research to seek out evidence to dispute this statement. However, it would be unwise to assume that there are no elements of professional self-interest and nurse-centredness present in the use of either the nursing process or patient allocation. Certainly, members of other professions (notably medicine) have articulated some alarm at these recent developments in the delivery of care (e.g. Mitchell, 1984). Influential nurses, on the other hand, have supported the notion of independence (Pembrey, 1983).

In the long term, it may be necessary to define those aspects of the nursing process and patient allocation that are 'nurse-' or 'patient'-centred, and at the same time be able to distinguish which elements of these two separate entities are advantageous or disadvantageous to the other dimension.

Although this section of the literature review has examined briefly the relationship between the nursing process/patient allocation and professionalism, the research itself will concentrate on the relevance of patient allocation to patient-centredness, bearing in mind the importance of nurse-centredness.

Having discussed the general confusion that surrounds the terminology used to describe the structure and function of work organisation, it would be helpful to look at some specific definitions of certain structural terms relating to work organisation, which enjoy popular contemporary currency. Hunt and Marks-Maran (1980) have provided the following glossary:

- *Task allocation*: the assignment of individual jobs to a particular nurse.
- *Team nursing*: the organisation of staff into teams of nurses led by a staff nurse or senior student. The team leader is responsible for planning the care that the team carries out using either a task or patient allocation system of work.
- *Patient allocation*: each nurse is responsible for the care of a small group of patients.

Hunt and Marks-Maran also discuss variations of patient allocation, e.g. a nurse being allocated to a patient for one span of duty only, or for up to the whole length of patient stay.

The authors did not state how the care of the patient was catered for when the allocated nurse was off duty. Was the patient 'shadow-allocated' to just one other person, or were many different nurses involved in his or her care? There is much made of the notion of 'continuity of care' in the professional ideology. Metcalfe (1982, p.376) noted that:

> 'for the patients, "individualised care" did not necessarily necessitate "continuity of care"; the majority of mothers did enjoy having the same nurses and midwives coming back to care for them. Because nurses and midwives are not on duty all day, every day, perfect continuity of care for hospital patients is an unrealistic ideal.'

Marks-Maran (1978, p.413) asserted that:

> 'Patient allocation can be used in a modified way without the Nursing Process but the Nursing Process cannot function without a system of patient allocation.'

This notion is debatable, since it could be perfectly feasible, given the traditional method of work organisation (task allocation), that phases of the nursing process could be task allocated – indeed, many present-day ward sisters would argue that they have been using the nursing process for a long time, i.e. assessing the patient's needs, planning the care, delegating the implementation of the care, usually by tasks in a hierarchical order, and, finally, monitoring the results of the care and redefining further needs. However, this approach leaves most of the power and accountability for care decisions in the hands of the sister, while the rest of the staff carry out and are accountable for fragments of care.

A more recent sophistication of patient allocation (which also probably reflects a more realistic structure in which the nursing process can function, particularly if the primary nurse is qualified or at least a senior student) is primary nursing, which Grant (1979, p.35) describes as:

> 'a modification of patient assignment in which one nurse is responsible for the planning and evaluation of the care of certain patients, other nurses are responsible for the giving of that care when the primary nurse is off duty. The patient knows who his nurse is. The

nurse, too, is in a better position to know "her" patients and thus to help plan their care; a consistency can therefore be provided which might be lacking in other systems of allocation.'

The author points out that primary nursing should not be confused with the term 'primary care', which refers to the initial assessment, diagnosis and treatment of nursing needs.

The literature tends to support the Briggs assertion that the dominant practice of work organisation in hospital wards is one orientated towards task allocation. Bendall (1975), in her research in 20 training schools, suggested that task allocation was the norm in the hospitals that she studied. She also argued that patient-centred care had never been practised.

Despite Bendall's pessimism regarding the incidence of patient allocation, other researchers have located this practice, albeit in limited forms. Hawthorn (1974), in her study of nine paediatric wards, was able to locate just one ward practising patient allocation. Pembrey (1975), using a sample of 50 ward sisters, found nine of them who were said to be organising the work in such a way as to produce individualised care.

THE ORGANISATION OF NURSING WORK

The most recently known study into the organisation of nursing work is that by Metcalfe (1982). She offered more plausible explanations for the rare practice of patient allocation, in terms of staff shortages and the departure of the original instigator of the scheme.

Metcalfe discussed at some length the work of Auld (1968), Boekholdt and Kanters (1978) and Chavasse (1976), which she found did not 'provide evidence to support the reputed advantages'. Metcalfe, herself, hoped also to carry out an experimental study into the reputed advantages of patient allocation, using a more rigorous research design.

Unfortunately, despite this increased rigour, she, too, was unable to produce evidence to support the suggested advantages of patient allocation, and, although she acknowledged the confusion surrounding the terms 'patient allocation' and 'nursing process', the study does little to disentangle this.

Metcalfe acknowledged that task allocation might not

necessarily mean bad care, but did not suggest why this might be. She did, however, clarify the issue a little, when she later stated:

'A ward sister or charge nurse who is willing to introduce a system of patient allocation on to her/his ward is often a person who is interested in improving standards of care, interested in providing opportunities for learners and who is likely to have progressive ideas. Such a person is likely to ensure good patient care regardless of the system used to organise the work.' (p.22)

Although Metcalfe was implying the importance of the role of the ward sister in relation to good care, she did not enlarge on how this was achieved, apart from by the willingness on the part of the sister to introduce patient allocation. She did, however, make an important passing reference to the weakness inherent in the argument of relating the development of individualised care to the structure that was believed to have produced it. She went on to question this assumption in view of recent research:

'Patient allocation, by virtue of the structural arrangements made to deliver care, is associated with individualised care. The invariability of this association can be questioned in the light of the conclusions drawn from a recent research study (Luker, 1980). Luker suggested that it was the *interpersonal* processes involved in the delivery of care which "individualised" otherwise standard interventions.' (Metcalfe, 1982, p.14)

Clearly, it is important to distinguish between 'structural arrangements' and 'interpersonal processes'. This current study will concentrate on the latter.

Unfortunately, Metcalfe's experimental research design, which involved monitoring patient and staff satisfaction levels in a maternity ward before and after the introduction of patient allocation, failed to identify these interpersonal processes. In her main conclusion, she suggested that future research should concentrate on developing 'a method of assessing the quality of nursing care given on wards which have been graded as to their "degree of patient centredness"' (pp.371–372).

It has become clear from this current research that it is of crucial importance for the nursing profession to discriminate between notions of:

- patient-centredness and patient allocation; and
- task-centredness and task allocation.

Then it will be in a position to make an informed provision of nursing care, and to understand how nurses can influence the nature of the patient's experience of the hospital world.

THE CARE OF CHILDREN IN HOSPITAL

As a consequence of the Platt Report (1959), Stacey et al (1970) investigated the difficulties of implementing the Platt recommendations, particularly those regarding open visiting, mothers-in and attendant problems. This literature pointed out that:

> '[the nurse's] relationship with the patient is basically discontinuous and fragmentary since, like any other person providing a specialised service, she is present only when the curative process demands her specialised ministrations ... the nurse has little opportunity for emotional involvement with the patient.' (p.112)

The latter point is explained by increased patient turnover, staff shortages and the changing philosophy of nurse education. The mode of work organisation was not monitored as a possible contributory factor.

The Stacey et al (1970) data also showed that the amount of interaction that individual children had with the nursing staff was extremely low (e.g. half an hour per day) and, in fact, some children were alone and unoccupied for up to 80% of their waking hours. It was felt that this could be exacerbated by the fact that children are not mature enough to provide each other with the emotional support that adults frequently contribute in the hospital situation.

Stacey et al's work was further supported by evidence from research by Cleary (1977), who looked at the distribution of nursing attention in a children's ward. She found that task allocation was the mode of work organisation, and, by the use of activity sampling, it was found that learners provided 75% of recorded contacts with the children, but that they did not make the most of these contacts to interact socially with the children. (The Briggs Report [1972] also stated that learners provided 75% of all nursing care.) Because task allocation was practised, it was felt that there were too many people involved in the care of the children, which produced less attention and a blindness to individual needs; care was fragmented and nurses did not notice, and, therefore, did not relieve, overt distress.

A study by Hall (1977) described the introduction of play leaders into children's wards. As a result of this innovation, the children became more mobile, which in turn produced greater activity and communication with others.

Hall and Stacey (1979) provided fresh evidence and expanded on earlier work by offering a psychosocial view of children's encounters with illness and hospitals. Jacobs (1979, in Hall and Stacey) discussed the denial of emotions in the ward setting. She examined the way in which professionalisation of specialisation in Western medicine had encouraged fragmentation of care, to the extent that the emotional aspects of the illness experience might be underplayed or even denied. She asserted that staff must themselves receive psychosocial support if they are to invest psychosocially in the patients and in each other.

Jacobs goes on to discuss many social structures that she feels facilitate the depersonalisation of the patient, including the routinisation of the nursing work using a task-centred approach.

In the same publication (Hall and Stacey, 1979), Cleary, in her chapter on the effects of the style of work allocation on the distribution of nursing attention, noted that:

> 'It became apparent that the way in which the work of the nurses was organised had important implications for the care of child patients.' (p.109)

She graphically described situations of intense distress in a children's ward, which was essentially task orientated in the organisation of the nursing work. Cleary (1979) concluded that changes in both orientation and work organisation were necessary to reduce the distress of hospitalisation for child patients.

It has been suggested that children's needs would become more apparent if there was a less discontinuous view of them, and that patient assignment might provide for this. It was also argued that quality of care using this system might also be improved, by being less fragmented, with more sociable interaction provided by a smaller number of nurses interacting with any one child. These research studies appear to confirm the professional ideology in relation to the negative aspects of task allocation. They also reflect the views of the profession in relation to the assumed advantages of a patient allocation system of work organisation.

NURSING RESEARCH ON CHILDREN IN HOSPITAL

Nursing research into the quality of nursing care in relation to sick children is meagre. However, Hawthorn's (1974) study of nine paediatric units does make a valuable and considerable contribution to an area of study that has largely been neglected by nurse researchers. She claimed that little was known about what nurses actually did in children's wards. Hawthorn's study was grounded on the assumption that nursing care of an acceptable quality could only exist if the total needs of the patient (psychosocial and physical) were acknowledged and met.

The study sought to replicate work carried out by Pill (1970), who found that nurse–patient interaction was low and was usually associated with the delivery of routine care, of which play was not a feature. The nurses appeared to resent the presence of parents and, in one hospital, the nurses actually restricted the visiting.

Hawthorn's (1974) work tended to support the findings made by Pill (1970), and, although Hawthorn did not focus specifically on work organisation, she included questions relating to this in her questionnaire to nursing staff. The questionnaire itself was structured around the recommendations made by Platt in 1959. In Hawthorn's sample of nine paediatric units, only one was said to practise case assignment.

Hawthorn suggested that the root of the problem of providing high quality care lay in the numbers of nurses interacting with the children, and that, by reducing the numbers of nurses interacting, it would be possible to try different methods of delivering care and, thereby, improving it. She made no mention of the importance of patient-centredness as a contrast to task-centredness, regardless of the numbers of staff interacting.

Hawthorn (1974) concluded that there had been very little improvement in the care of sick children since the publication of the Platt Report (1959). Her main recommendation concerned staff development in relation to current child-care theories. She believed that this would enable nurses to make appropriate changes to ward organisation.

Hawthorn continued to imply that changes in the structure in which care was given would lead to improvement in that care, particularly in relation to the care of child patients.

STANDARDS OF NURSING CARE

A recurring thread throughout the narrative so far has been notions of standards of care. There is a very real difficulty in defining these. Nevertheless, this difficulty should not preclude a constructive confrontation of such important issues. Lelean (1980, p.93) stated that:

'Research into nursing practice is hampered to a large extent by a lack of objective criteria against which to measure standards of care.'

Evers (1984) referred to the immense body of literature relating to standards of care emerging from North America from the late 1950s onward. She also noted the Royal College of Nursing's studies in the late 1960s, which looked at specific aspects of care, including the development of indices of quality. Despite these studies, Evers (1984, pp.48–49) concluded that:

'the fundamental problem of all measures of patient care remains, not surprisingly, unresolved: how to define "ideal" patient care in terms of which actual care and its outcomes can be assessed. Thus a major drawback of most measures is that they embody assumptions which are perhaps untestable, about the outcomes of particular nursing practices for patients.'

Evers went on to examine current measures to improve standards of care, such as the QUALPACS scale (Wandelt and Ager, 1974), in current use at Burford Hospital in Oxfordshire (Wainwright and Burnip, 1983). As a result of this examination, Evers concluded that:

'There is little concrete evidence, then, that so-called measures of patient care standards are much good or much use.' (p.59)

Evers (1984), in her research on geriatric patients' experiences, decided to rely on the notion that it is easier to arrive at a consensus definition of concrete instances of poor rather than 'ideal' care. Despite this rather gloomy view, the nursing profession continues to be preoccupied with standards of care.

The Royal College of Nursing's (1980) discussion document *Standards of Nursing Care* suggested that care can be evaluated in three dimensions: *structure* – external conditions necessary for the activity of nursing to take place, e.g. environment or administrative policies; *process* – what is done and how it is performed;

and *outcome* – the results of nursing activity in terms of its effect on the patient. Paragraph 45 of the document goes on to state that:

> 'Structure evaluation in terms of standards of care has predominated to date. This is not altogether surprising for it is comparatively easier and less threatening to staff to quantify personnel and duration of activities rather than to examine and question standards of practice. Yet until standards of practice in the qualitative components are established and measured, structure evaluation may be based on invalid assumptions of acceptable care levels.'

The RCN document does not suggest how the qualitative components of care might be established. However, it might be helpful at this point to remind ourselves of Metcalfe's (1982) views in relation to this problem. She believed that it would be useful to measure quality of care in terms of patient-centredness, because care that was individualised would, 'by definition, be improved' (p.372).

Clearly, there are many pitfalls that can be anticipated in defining criteria for patient-centredness, not least in relation to subjective value judgments about what constitutes patient-centred care. Concern could also be expressed regarding ethical and moral issues – how is a nurse to demonstrate 'patient-centredness' when a patient says, 'Let me die'? Alongside these issues are more complex considerations concerning the nature of the patient, his or her state of health, the physical and psycho-social environment and, finally, the nature of nursing itself. These considerations are currently being addressed by professional nurses in their quest to provide a theoretical base to nursing care.

However, the notion of establishing criteria for patient-centredness has much to recommend it in the absence of other, less problematic approaches to the qualitative evaluation of standards of care.

SUMMARY

This literature review began by examining the notion that a patient allocation system of work organisation would improve standards of nursing care, and would be particularly appropriate for the delivery of nursing care to sick children. However, the proliferation of terms used to describe different approaches to nursing care has tended to confuse rather than clarify the structure, process and function dimensions of nursing activity. This has been further complicated by the difficulty of defining 'good care' in qualitative terms, leading Evers (1984, p.51) to assert that it is easier to agree about 'concrete instances of bad or unacceptable care'.

In recent years, the assumed advantages of patient allocation have been transferred wholesale to the nursing process, which is also associated with overt notions of professionalism. Research into the organisation of nursing (Auld, 1968; Boekholdt and Kanters, 1978; Chavasse, 1981; Metcalfe, 1982) have been inconclusive in relation to supporting the assumed advantages to the patient of a patient allocation system.

Research into the care of children in hospital (Stacey et al, 1970; Hawthorn, 1974; Hall, 1977; Hall and Stacey, 1979) has shown that hospitals were distressing to sick children. Although the most recent research located was reported in 1979, two more recent publications by the Consumers' Association (1980, 1985) suggest that hospitals continue to be distressing places for sick children. Both reports had been concerned mainly with the provision of special facilities for sick children, e.g. wards for children only, open visiting, residential parents and provision of care by specially trained staff.

The 1980 report expressed the view that some children showed a lack of trust in the nurses, and that this might have been avoided if care had been more individualised or nurse–patient relationships had been allowed to develop. There was evidence to suggest that staff believed that developing relationships could be detrimental (to what or whom?): 'Better than getting too involved'.

2 | Research methodology

INTRODUCTION

Dingwall and McIntosh (1978) maintain that British nursing research methodology has adopted a scientistic rather than a naturalistic approach. They argue that the latter is more appropriate because it views people as independent beings with freewill, capable of making choices. They go on to criticise the more narrow interpretation of the concept of scientific inquiry in terms of mathematical logic, as they felt that this should be broadened to include a questioning mind, demonstrating a healthy scepticism.

Dingwall and McIntosh (1978, p.12) concluded:

> 'When we are asking questions of quantity, "how many, how fast, how great a proportion", then we need to use methods which give quantitative answers, but as soon as we start to ask more complex questions, about why a certain state of affairs should be so, then we need a different sort of research.'

It was believed that the 'naturalistic' approach was pertinent to this present study, the purpose of which was to investigate whether there was any relationship between patterns of work organisation and various outcomes for sick children, with particular reference to the popular notion that a patient allocation type of work organisation has the potential to confront some of the negative outcomes in the ward environment.

It was felt that the research problem, which focused on three categories of ward participants – the ward sister, the nurses and the patients – demanded a variety of research methods in order to cover adequately the issues involved.

Burgess (1982) drew attention to various writers who had suggested different methods of checking validity and avoiding narrowness in social research methodology. Stacey (1969) suggested 'combined operations', Denzin (1970) proposed 'triangulation' and Douglas (1976) suggested 'mixed strategies'.

Burgess (1982) attempts to synthesise these different ideas using the notion of 'multiple strategies', which he sees as a means of overcoming 'the problems of the single-method, single-investigator, single-data, single-theory study'. However, he acknowledges that the use of multiple strategies could be extremely expensive in terms of time and money.

Spencer (1983) reinforces the earlier criticism of Dingwall and McIntosh (1978) of the current tendency in nursing research to adopt a positivist theoretical position. He argues that this approach 'treats people as objects', and that researchers of nursing should 'search for a different and more human research method'.

Lazarsfeld and Barton (1971) argue that systematic study in the social sciences can be achieved by various devices, which may not include 'strict quantitative measurement' but which are superior to 'unaided individual judgment'.

Clearly, despite the fact that one is unable to be totally objective, it is possible to achieve varying degrees of rigour, the greater the better. Lundberg (1971) introduces a note of caution in terms of the existence of observer bias in all areas of study, which can be reduced by the use of different research tools and the discipline of scientific training.

Scientific rigour may also be facilitated by the use of both research and methodological triangulation. Since the financial resources of this present study did not stretch to the use of several researchers from different backgrounds using different approaches, the use of multiple strategies became more important and enabled a great deal of cross-checking to take place. Perhaps Schatzman and Strauss (1973, p.ix) should be allowed the final word in relation to strategies for a natural sociology:

> 'The general and immediate interests of the researcher are broadly scientific; that is, the researcher is interested primarily in describing, understanding and explaining the activities of his hosts.'

To some degree, the choice of research methods was influenced by the techniques used by Hall (1975) in his comparative longitudinal study, which examined the introduction of a play leader scheme to the children's wards in two hospitals. The research design used by Hall seemed to go part way to answering the criticism levelled by Spencer (1983) at the methodology of nursing research, in that Hall focused on the interactive processes that went on between the hospital staff, the children and the play leaders.

These methods appeared to be successful and were, therefore, useful when constructing the present research design, which sought to extend the qualitative nature of the data, particularly in relation to the study of the ward sister. The emphasis of Hall's (1975) research lay on the introduction of play leaders and how they related to changes in work organisation and social relations in the ward setting. This present study concentrates on how the ward sisters' deployment of the work force affects the experiences of the sick children. It was, therefore, important to take into account this change in emphasis from play leaders to ward sisters in the subsequent research design. By initially carrying out observations in two wards that were said to practise different methods of work organisation, the aim was to identify and explain any differences in patients' experiences. Because of the paucity of research in this particular area, it was decided to adopt an in-depth exploratory case study approach in just two wards. This approach has been defined by Foreman (1971, p.184):

'a method of organising data for the purpose of analysing the life of a social unit – a person, a family, a culture group or even an entire community.'

Clamp (1984), in her justification for a case-study approach in the fields of social science and nursing education, makes the point that quantitative approaches to the exploration of the complexities of human behaviour in equally complicated settings is not always possible, and that qualitative data enable a more appropriate and equally valid examination to be made. Clamp goes on to outline the work done by the Nuffield Foundation in response to suspicions about the value of a case study approach:

'Because suspicions persisted the Nuffield Foundation organised an international conference in Cambridge in 1975 to consider the whole subject (Adelman et al, 1975). The possible advantages of this type of research were identified as follows:

case studies were strong in reality and generalisations could be made
about elements described
the complexity of social situations was recognised
an archive of descriptive material was obtained which was
sufficiently rich to permit subsequent re-interpretation
contributions to an evolving situation were made
findings were more publicly accessible in the sense that the language
and form of presentation was less dependent upon specialised
interpretation.' (pp.78–79)

Yin (1984) claims that the case-study approach enables the
researcher to capture 'the holistic and meaningful characteristics
of real life events' at all levels of human activity.

In the light of these discussions, it was considered that a case-
study approach was appropriate for this current research.

The research methods to be described are as follows:

1. open-ended observation of admissions;
2. time-sampled observation of child case studies for the first 4
    days of admission or until discharge (whichever was the
    shorter period);
3. diary records of the child case studies following the time-
    sampled observations;
4. time-sampled observations of ward activities;
5. continuous open-ended observations of the two ward sisters
    for whole spans of duty for a period of 3 days;
6. semi-structured interviews with the ward sisters.

Methods 2, 3 and 4 were modified from Hall's (1975) research. The
interview schedule was based on one used by Pembrey (1978) for
her research into the role of the ward sister in relation to
individualised patient care. The method of observation used to
study the ward sister and the admission process is common to
many field researchers operating in a variety of settings. This has
usually entailed the researcher writing up observations retro-
spectively (Wax, 1971), but in this current study, observations
were recorded in situ.

Fox (1966) acknowledges that while direct observation can
introduce distortion, this can be neutralised by a period of
acclimatisation and orientation.

Before describing the research methods in detail, a pen portrait
of the two study wards will be given, in order to contextualise the
interactional scenario.

THE CHILDREN'S WARDS

As Hawthorn (1974) points out, there is no official data base from which it is possible to identify wards that are using different styles of work organisation. It was, therefore, via an informal professional network that these two wards were located as allegedly practising, on the one hand, patient allocation, and on the other, task allocation.

Both wards formed part of the hospital's medical unit and were, therefore, under the nursing administrative jurisdiction of the same nursing officer. Although the geographical layout of the wards was very similar, the ward that was said to practise patient allocation had 20 beds and cots, while the ward said to practise task allocation had only 17 beds and cots. This deficit on the task allocation ward was created by part of the floor space being taken up by a special day care unit, which was not included in the study. Since patients in this unit tended to be day cases and were cared for by a full-time special unit sister, it was necessary for the main ward staff to become involved only if a child required an overnight stay, which was very rare. This lower bed/cot capacity on the task allocation ward contributed, to some extent, to a lower work load than that experienced on the patient allocation ward. Added to this was the fact that the patient allocation ward had more consultant staff attached to it; the patient turnover was also more rapid on the patient allocation ward, which had slightly lower staffing levels to cope with the resultant increase in patients. The 'busy-ness factors' of each ward are discussed in more detail in chapter 3. Both wards provided training facilities for nursing students.

Although both wards belonged to the same medical unit, the conditions for which they catered were intrinsically different. The patient allocation ward cared mainly for children suffering from malignancies and renal or haematological disorders. The children's medical care was overseen by six consultants. The permanent nursing staff consisted of a senior and junior ward sister, two full-time and one part-time staff nurse, two state enrolled nurses and two auxiliary nurses (all full-time), a part-time ward clerk, a full-time sister responsible for haemophilia patients and a part-time oncology staff nurse. (The last two nurses had some peripatetic functions, e.g. out-patients clinics, home visits etc., and thus were not continuously present.)

The task allocation ward cared for children suffering from endocrine, neurological and respiratory disorders. There were four consultants to oversee the children's medical care. The permanent nursing staff consisted of a senior and a junior sister, three full-time staff nurses, one full-time nursery nurse, two full-time auxiliaries, one part-time auxiliary, two part-time state enrolled nurses and a full-time ward clerk. Both wards catered for children from the age of 12 months to 16 years.

RESEARCH METHODS

The child studies

It was proposed that 10 children on each ward would be observed 'in depth' from the point of admission, and for up to 4 days or until discharge, depending on which occurred earlier. The size of the sample was determined by the time available and the fact that the researcher was working alone. However, it was believed that these in-depth studies would provide sufficient evidence to establish degrees of child-centredness on each ward.

Since the researcher wished to be present when the child was admitted, to observe how the admission procedure was handled by the staff, it was necessary for the researcher to be available throughout the whole of the first day (usually Monday) of each weekly research schedule, in order to observe two admissions, if possible, before the time-sampled observations commenced at 17.00 hrs. These observations continued until 22.00 hrs (with a break for supper at 19.00 hrs), in order to cover the child's first evening in hospital, during which the parents would have left the child, possibly for the first time, totally in the care of the staff. This time could often be stressful for the child, and it was important to observe how the staff cared for him or her.

The admissions

Both wards had only a limited number of planned admissions; the majority of admissions were unplanned and could arrive at any time of the day or night. It was, therefore, decided to make the age range fairly broad, in order to obtain the requisite number of cases in the time available. The age range included those children who had started school but were pre-pubescent, i.e. 5 to 10 years of age. Despite the breadth of the age range and the decision not to take other variables into account, there were some occasions when no suitable admissions occurred or when there was only one admission; there was one notable instance when the researcher waited for 3 days, to no avail.

Verbal consent was obtained from the parents of the children selected for observation after they had been given details of the project; letters with information about the project were available on the ward for parents of the other children. The researcher was always willing to discuss the project with any parents who expressed an interest in what was happening.

Initially the admission of the child was observed by recording in situ open-ended observations, which focused on the interaction between the nurse and the family unit. The observations, on the whole, commenced with the arrival of the family on the ward and were discontinued when, in the researcher's opinion, the admission procedure was deemed to have been completed. It was

Table 1 Patient allocation ward: children observed

	Sex	Observation period	Age	Diagnosis
1. Nigel	Male	4 days	9 yr 2 mnth	Acute myeloid leukaemia
2. Suleiman	Male	2 days	7 yr	Upper respiratory tract infection, ?meningitis
3. Sandhu	Male	4 days	5 yr 1 mnth	Haemophilia
4. Lesley	Female	4 days	7 yr 4 mnth	Nephrotic syndrome
5. Margaret	Female	4 days	7 yr 3 mnth	Astrocytoma of cerebellum
6. Billy	Male	3 days	7 yr 10 mnth	Renal investigations
7. Caroline	Female	4 days	8 yr 5 mnth	For stabilisation of hypertension. Nephrectomy
8. Sarah	Female	3 days	7 yr 2 mnth	Haematuria
9. Balbinder	Female	4 days	8 yr	Painful swollen joints
10. Amanda	Female	2 days	6 yr	Haematuria
11. James	Male	4 days	9 yr 4 mnth	Acute asthmatic attack

Table 2 Task allocation ward: children observed

	Sex	Observation period	Age	Diagnosis
1. Surinder	Female	3 days	9 yr 2 mnth	Investigation of congenital heart disease. ?Cerebral abscess
2. Shirley	Female	4 days	10 yr 5 mnth	Cystic fibrosis for i.v. therapy
3. Arnold	Male	4 days	5 yr 1 mnth	Right orbital cellulitis
4. Emily	Female	4 days	8 yr 11 mnth	Investigation of immune deficiency
5. Patrick	Male	2 days	8 yr 1 mnth	Croup
6. Laurie	Male	4 days	9 yr 3 mnth	Asthma
7. Maralyn	Female	4 days	10 yr 3 mnth	Abdominal pain. 'Ataxia'
8. Jenny	Female	4 days	9 yr 1 mnth	Spastic quadraplegia due to cerebral anoxia
9. Ronald	Male	4 days	6 yr 4 mnth	Diabetes
10. Paul	Male	4 days	4 yr	Lobar pneumonia
11. Shah	Male	4 days	8 yr 4 mnth	Chest infection, ?TB

important for this to take place before 17.00 hrs when the time-sampled observations were scheduled to begin.

At the end of the data collection period, 11 children on each ward had been observed in detail. Tables 1 and 2 show the ages and disease categories of the samples of children observed on each ward. Both sets of data reflect very accurately the disease categories of the total child population of the wards, and could, therefore, be said to be fairly representative of the conditions being treated and cared for by the nursing staff.

The ward study
Figure 1 shows the half-hourly observation schedule. It will be noted that the first 10 minutes were allocated to the compilation of a ward study. This entailed the researcher moving through the ward in a predetermined order and recording on the ward study observation sheet (figure 2, p.26) the position, activity and mood of each child (including the detailed case study children).

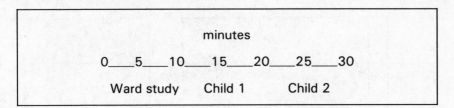

minutes

0___5___10___15___20___25___30

Ward study   Child 1   Child 2

Figure 1 Half-hourly observation schedule

Additionally, the identity of interactors was established; if possible, a note was made in relation to the content or reason for the interaction. An observation code was used to record these items (figure 3, p.27). The same code was used for the individual child studies. Although these observations were child focused, they did take into account other social actors present on the ward, e.g. parents, nurses, school teachers, etc.

Since the study was also concerned with what the nurses did, and as it was likely that the nurses might sometimes be doing something other than interacting with the children, it was necessary to include a separate ward study sheet (figure 4, p.28) in order to establish what the nursing staff were doing when not interacting with the children.

This would provide a picture not only of what the staff did when not with the children, but also of how much movement of staff around the ward there was. It was, therefore, quite possible for the same nurse to be recorded several times with different children on the children's ward study sheets, and also for her to be 'sighted' interacting with different colleagues, thus also being recorded on the ward study staff sheet.

The children
Each pair of case study children was observed in detail for 5 minutes each (see figure 1). Each 5 minutes was divided into 10-second intervals with the use of a stopwatch and the same codes were employed as for the ward study.

The observation sheet (figure 5, p.29), besides being divided into 10-second intervals, had an upper large rectangular area for long-hand comments. The top, smaller rectangle was used for noting who the social interactors were, and the upper and lower triangular spaces for recording position and mood/activity level respectively.

DATE: Monday

Child: Ann Setlin   **Age**: 6 years   **Diagnosis**: Cystic fibrosis

	1	2	3	4	5	6	7	8
TIME	5.00p.m.	5.30p.m.	6.00p.m.	6.30p.m.	8.00p.m.	8.30p.m.	9.00p.m.	9.30p.m.
POSITION	B							
ACTIVITY	3							
WITH	P.V.							
MOOD	C							
EXTRA	Lying quietly in bed							
COMMENTS	Mum knitting							

Child: Mark Jones   **Age**: 4 years   **Diagnosis**: Asthma

	1	2	3	4	5	6	7	8
TIME								
POSITION								
ACTIVITY								
WITH								
MOOD								
EXTRA								
COMMENTS								

Figure 2 Ward study observation sheet (children)

Position

B   = Bed
OK   = On knee
CA   = Carried
U   = Up in chair
UA   = Up and about

Activity

1 = Asleep
2 = Awake, unobservant
3 = Awake, observant
4 = Active

Social actors

N   = Nurses
PV   = Parents/visitors
Drs = Doctors
OS   = Other staff
T/PL = Teacher/play leader

Mood

E = Excitedly happy
H = Happy
C = Contented
A = Apathetic
D = Distressed
P = Pandemonium distress

Figure 3 Observation code

This detailed 5-minute observation was followed by a 5-minute, long-hand diary account, which not only elaborated on what had occurred during the previous 5 minutes, but was also concerned with current activity.

Hall (1975) noted the criticism of time-sampling methods, that 'they invariably distort the flow of events by imposing arbitrary starting and finishing points (Wright, 1960; also Holt and Reynell, 1970)'. However, he considered the alternative for collecting quantitative descriptions of behaviour, in the form of event sampling, to be suitable mainly for the recording of infrequently occurring activities, and that the time-sampling technique could be made more flexible and, thus, less distortive, by not restricting the use of the 10-second interval to one initiative or response in the interactive process. He concluded that the method adopted was satisfactory for providing an interactional summary, because it 'reproduced the observed behaviour in considerable detail'.

Since this current research made the same demands of the time-sampling framework, Hall's approach was considered to be useful, and was, therefore, replicated with only minor modifications in relation to the number of coded categories, which was, in fact, reduced.

As with Hall's (1975) study and the earlier Swansea work (Pill, 1970), it was found that a maximum of 4 hours for observation periods was a reasonable limit for any one observer, to avoid the

Nursing staff: Task allocation ward

Position:

Activity with: N, PV, T/PL, OS, Dr
(when nurse is not interacting with patient)
øNurse not seen

Nursing staff on duty	Duty time	Time							
		5.00p.m. 1	5.30p.m. 2	6.00p.m. 3	6.30p.m. 4	8.00p.m. 5	8.30p.m. 6	9.00p.m. 7	9.30p.m. 8
Sister Smith	Late	Doing drugs with N. Palfrey							
N. Palfrey	Late	See above							
N. Jones	Late	Talking to Simon Phipps, etc.							
A/N Brown	Late	Doing drinks							
NIGHT STAFF							——— ON DUTY		
Late shift: 12.45p.m. to 9.30p.m.									
Other people on the ward not included in the ward study		R.C. Priest talking to James and Mother. Doctor in treatment room alone							

Figure 4 Ward study observation sheet (staff)

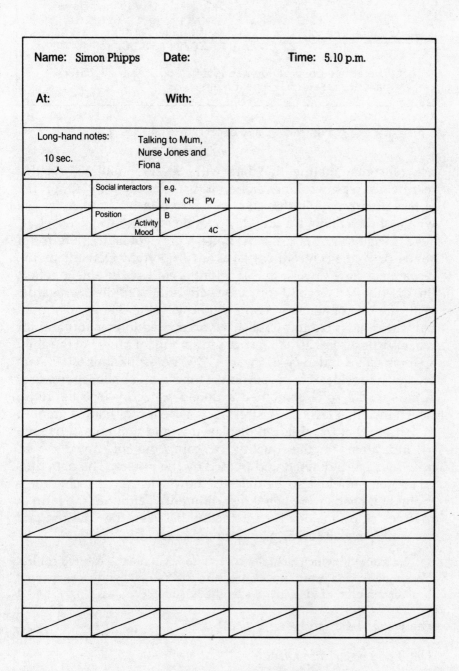

Figure 5 Individual child study observation sheet

	Day 1	Day 2	Day 3	Day 4
Observation period	17.00 hrs	06.30 hrs	10.00 hrs	12.00 hrs
	23.00 hrs	11.30 hrs	13.00 hrs	17.00 hrs

N.B. The above observation periods include 1 hour allocated
daily for researcher meal breaks.

Figure 6   Daily observation periods

risk of contaminating the data with observer fatigue. As this
researcher was working alone, it was decided to adopt the
observation schedule depicted in figure 6 in order to cover the
whole of the child's waking day over days of the week.

As in Hall's (1975) thesis, the pattern of negotiation, in terms of
child- or nurse-centredness, was an important element of the
research design. It was necessary for the codes to be able to reflect
the distribution of child- or nurse-centredness in the two wards.
With the use of codes in conjunction with the diaries, it should
have been possible to establish who initiated interaction and for
what purpose, and also to record the amount of time that the child
spent inactive and awake. Cleary (1979) notes that this latter state
took up a considerable proportion of time in a task allocation ward.
Although the code contained a 'mood' category (see figure 3),
which included levels of distress, it was believed that the amount
of distress that the children displayed would not in itself be seen
as indicative of the quality of care, but of how it was
acknowledged, defined and treated by the nurses. The data thus
generated should also be able to show whether the children's
individual needs were being met differently, either in the form of
routines or by negotiative interaction between the children and
the staff. As Hall (1975, p.75) pointed out:

'The extent to which a child acquired information and exerted control
seemed to be a useful measure of the child's independence from the
determination of his activities by the hospital.'

The ward sister study

The 3-day observation study
The two ward sisters were observed for a total of 3 days each.
The first day of observation in both cases covered a Tuesday early

shift (07.45 hrs – 16.30 hrs). Each sister had Wednesday as an observation-free day. Then followed observation of a late shift on Thursday (13.00 hrs – 21.30 hrs) and another early shift on Friday. This was believed to be an improvement on Pembrey's (1978) research method (she observed each sister for one day only, but had over 50 sisters in her sample), as the increased length of observation time may have reduced the possibility of a 'halo' effect on the sisters' work performance or the observation of an unrepresentative day.

Neither ward sister knew until the first day of the observation when observations were to take place. Therefore, it was impossible for her to make any special plans with regard to the off-duty, etc. for this event. The ward sister study was also carried out after several child studies had been completed, so that the sisters had become accustomed to the presence of the researcher on their ward.

The research role adopted for the purpose of both the ward/child studies and the ward sister studies was not totally non-participatory, but rather of a 'participant as observer' nature. This is defined as a role in which both the observed and the observer are aware of the field relationship (Gold, 1971).

There are, of course, dangers associated with such a research role, which Gold quite rightly emphasises. These include the field worker 'going native', which clearly is a considerable risk in the case of a professional nurse carrying out nursing research in a clinical setting. The reverse may also happen, whereby the informant identifies too much with the field worker, so much so that the informing role changes to that of 'partner in observation'. Gold (1971) suggests that this situation might be overcome by maintaining certain boundaries of intimacy to sustain the notion of a 'sociological stranger', who is then able to withdraw from the relationship at an appropriate time.

It was hoped that the data generated by the ward sister studies would be helpful in describing and, thus, defining systems of patient and task allocation types of work organisation. It was also hoped to establish whether the sisters' interactional styles differed with both the patients and the staff, particularly in terms of patient- and task-centredness.

The interviews
The researcher spent 3 months on each of the two wards. At the end of the total 6-month period, both ward sisters were interviewed

independently about their work and ward management. It was felt that this timing was appropriate, as both sisters would be used to the researcher, who would have spent a considerable period on each ward. Therefore, responses were less likely to be guarded and circumspect. The interviews themselves were semi-structured and similar to those used by Pembrey (1978; see figure 7).

The main aims were to establish why the sisters managed their wards in the way they did and to obtain some clues as to how they conceptualised their work, in terms of tasks or patients.

Franklin and Osborne (1971) noted that the best way to ascertain people's feelings, motives and opinions is to ask them. Schatzman and Strauss (1973, p.77) elaborate on this further when they state that:

> 'While direct observation is the heart of field research, the interview must be used to provide context or meaning. Without this, much of the action seen appears as motion. Asking the actor what he is doing, and why, is a necessary corrective to unwarranted observer imputation and inference. We need him to tell us what it means to be professional on a career course, working in an institution, with a philosophy (we assume) underlying his operations.'

Both interviews were recorded by hand, and, in the case of the task allocation ward sister, the interview lasted approximately 1 hour. The interview with the patient allocation sister lasted 1 hour 45 minutes. She appeared to find it much easier to be articulate about her work than did the task allocation sister.

RESEARCH STRATEGY

The pilot study

All the research methods used in the main study were first tested and revised in a small pilot study. A period of 2 weeks was spent in a children's ward of a district general hospital, observing the activities of the children and the staff. This enabled the researcher to develop some expertise in observational and recording skills.

In the original research strategy, the first 10 minutes of the 30-minute observation schedule were intended to be used for a 5-minute ward study and for 5 minutes of questioning specific nurses about their interactions with the case study children. This

Area being explored	*Discussion with the sister*
1. The ward	Background data about the ward
2. The background of the sister	Background data about the sister
3. Changes in the ward. Organisational instability, 'control' factor	Changes that have affected the sister's work, the patients, the doctors, nurses' training policy
4. Work role	Sister's description of her job
5. Work priorities	What are the most important daily jobs for you to do? What would you be unhappy to leave out?
6. Resources and constraints, control factor	Can you run the ward as you like? What stops you?
7. Work organisation	How do you describe the nursing work? Describe a typical day
8. Work prescription	How do the nurses know what to do?
9. Work allocation, deployment pattern	How do the nurses work?
10. Patients' needs	How are the patients' special daily needs met?
11. Work accountability	How do you find out what work has been done? How do you check the nurses' work?
12. The nurses work/training control factor	How do you feel about the nurses you are allocated?
13. Areas of importance to the sister	Have you any comments? What do you like most about your job? What do you like least? Describe the ward looking at its best

Figure 7 Semi-structured interview schedule

was changed, in order that the first 10 minutes might be devoted entirely to the collection of the ward study data (see figures 2 and 4).

There were two reasons for this, the only major change. First, it became clear that nurses were irritated at being questioned by the researcher about their interaction with the case study children. This appeared to be exacerbated by the fact that they knew the researcher to be a nurse, and it was implied that it must, therefore, be clear to her why interaction was taking place. It was essential that the researcher was as unobtrusive as possible, and it was felt that this activity prevented this. Second, it became clear that the wards in the main study would be much busier than the district general hospital ward (which operated at a 50% capacity during the pilot study); thus, 5 minutes would probably be insufficient time in which to collect the ward study data. This, in fact, proved to be the case, and the change made to the schedule was, therefore, appropriate.

The main study

Access was gained to the main study hospital by initially discussing the research with the District Nursing Officer. Meetings were then arranged with the Divisional and Senior Nursing Officers who had specific responsibility for this particular hospital.

Following this, consultation took place with the unit's nursing officer, who was responsible for organising meetings between the researcher and the two ward sisters, who were subsequently seen individually. All the aforementioned personnel received an outline of the study.

Initially, the ward sisters were understandably rather dubious about having their ward management styles investigated, and much reassurance was needed and given regarding anonymity.

Before the fieldwork on each ward began, the researcher held several informal discussion sessions with the available ward staff, in order to ensure that they were aware of the reasons for the researcher's presence, and to clarify any misconceptions. There were also letters available on each ward for both the staff (those who had not attended a discussion session or had arrived on the ward after the research had commenced) and the parents of the 'general child population'.

As has already been mentioned, the parents of the individual children being studied were approached separately by the researcher, in order to obtain an informed verbal consent for their child to be observed. There were no refusals. The researcher did not wear a uniform or a white coat, as it was felt that this might create a form of unconscious, bureaucratic coercion in obtaining consent from the parents. (However, a name badge was worn in order to confirm the researcher's identity and to legitimate her presence.) The researcher made no secret of her previous status (that of nurse tutor) in the National Health Service, with either the parents of the staff, as it was felt that it would be easier to operate in a climate of honesty. This approach proved to be very rewarding, as the researcher was able to participate in nursing work when data was not being collected. This seemed crucial in the construction of a trusting relationship between the researcher and the staff. It was also important in sustaining researcher credibility in a professional environment.

SUMMARY

This chapter has mapped out the research strategies that were evolved for the purpose of examining the nature of social relationships between staff and patients in two children's wards, which used different styles of work organisation, i.e. task and patient allocation.

Methodological triangulation was considered to be important since the researcher was working alone (and was, thus, unable to exploit multidisciplinary investigator triangulation). This was achieved by the use of non-participant observation of different categories of the ward population in the form of diary records and time sampling; semi-structured interviews were also used.

This particular research design generated a large amount of data, which necessitated careful selection for analysis. It was, therefore, decided to exclude the general ward study data, i.e. the observations of all the children and all the staff. It was also impossible to analyse all the time-sampled observations, of up to 4 days, for all 22 of the case study children. It was decided to select two of these from each ward for an in-depth study. The remaining data (3-day ward sister study, interviews and admission studies) were fully utilised. However, for the purpose of this publication, the overall analysis of the admission studies is omitted (see Brown 1986).

3 The ward sisters

INTRODUCTION

In chapter 2, the collection of data in relation to the ward sisters' activities was described. An important component of the ward sister study was the use of semi-structured interviews with each of the sisters. In order that the sisters might feel more comfortable and at ease with the researcher, the interviews were carried out after the collection of the rest of the data. It was also felt that the responses that they made would be more realistic because the researcher had already observed them at work. However, for the purpose of this book, it was thought to be more useful to examine the sisters' work concepts as demonstrated in the interviews, and at the same time to report on how these concepts were put into practice during the 3-day ward sister study.

It was felt to be important to interview the sisters as well as to watch what they did, in order to effect a degree of data triangulation, which could then be used to cross-check the interpretations being made. Although the researcher had a nursing background and was, therefore, less likely to experience the same level of social discomfort as might researchers from other disciplines when observing in a clinical setting, the point made by Haralambos (1980) was well heeded. He stated that 'since it is not possible to enter the consciousness of others, there is no certainty that the meanings identified by the observer are those employed by the actors' (p.319).

The main aims of the interviews were to learn something of each sister's biography, to collect data about the wards, to establish how each sister defined her work organisation in terms of task and patient allocation, and, finally and most importantly, to establish how they conceptualised their work in terms of patient- and task-centredness.

Systematic observations of how the ward sisters worked were made, starting about 1 month after the child studies had begun. A long-hand record was made of (as far as possible) everything that the sisters said or did, and note was made of the identity of everyone with whom they were interacting. The observations were not coded in any way. The long-hand notes were transcribed in full.

THE WARD SISTER STUDY

The transcripts were analysed in terms of two major categories of interaction, according to the direction of the interaction, i.e. interactions initiated by the sisters with others and interactions initiated by others with the sisters. These two major categories were further sub-divided, according to the reason for the 'sister-' or 'other-' initiated interactions. These sub-categories, with their definitions, are listed below.

1. *Basic information* This included any interaction concerned with the basic care of the patient, normally related to universal needs, e.g. hygiene, nutrition, elimination.
2. *Technical information* Interactions in this category were usually concerned with the medical treatment that the patient was receiving and were often, therefore, related to the disease category to which the patient had been medically designated.
3. *Sociable interaction* Examples of this included chatting, joking and playing.
4. *Psychosocial support* This category of interaction was related to actual or potential psychosocial distress and was usually initiated by the recipient of the support.
5. *Administration and housekeeping* This category of interaction involved any activity relating to the organisation or management of the ward and the maintenance of a hygienic/safe environment.
6. *Miscellaneous* This grouping included any interaction that did not fit any of the previously discussed categories.
7. *Content unknown* It was felt to be important to include this

category to reduce the 'miscellaneous' section. It was usually used for one-sided conversations, such as telephone calls, when the identity of the caller was unknown and the content or context of the interaction was not immediately apparent.

By consigning the interactors to groups, e.g. nurses or children, it became possible to construct a quantitative table indicating with whom the the sisters interacted and how often (see figures 8 and 9 below). It was also possible to show the content of the interactions by using the above categories, e.g. technical, sociable. Figure 10 below shows the content of the interaction between the sisters and the learner nurses.

These figures will be examined in more detail later. It should be noted that the percentages in the figures have been rounded upwards for 0.5% and above. Percentages below 0.5% have been rounded down. It is, therefore, possible for some aggregated percentages not to add up to the total percentage.

THE INTERVIEWS

Both sisters were asked to give facts about the ward. Although both wards were very similar in geographical layout and belonged to the same nursing unit for administrative purposes, the differences concerned the important variable of work-load. Evidence of this is visible in the interviews. The patient allocation ward had 20 beds and cots under the care of six consultants. In the interview, the patient allocation sister drew attention to the fact that previously there had been three consultants and one honorary consultant, but now there were five consultants and one honorary consultant. She said that this change had quadrupled the work-load in terms of referrals, ward rounds and extra liaising.

On the other hand, the task allocation ward had 17 beds and cots, with only four consultants. Examination of the patient admission figures during the data collection period for each ward presents further evidence of 'busy-ness factors'. The task allocation ward had 578 admissions over a 7-month period, compared to 807 on the patient allocation ward over the same period.

Of course, 'busy-ness factors' would be considerably affected by the number of staff available to care for the children. However, on the examination of staffing numbers, the task allocation ward not only had fewer children to care for, but also more staff to care for them. This ward appeared to have a full-time nursery nurse, a part-time auxiliary and a part-time equivalent staff nurse in excess of the staff available on the patient allocation ward.

Length of the stay of the children was not examined in detail, but from impressions gained during the data collection, it would appear that, on the whole, length of stay on the patient allocation ward was relatively short for rather more acutely ill children, while the task allocation ward appeared to care for longer-stay, more chronically ill children. (An Asian girl with Batten's Disease – manifested by mental retardation and spastic paralysis – had been an in-patient continuously for 9 years!) The individual child studies would appear to support the above impressions, although, of course, the samples are very small. However, in terms of disease, they do appear to be reasonably representative of the child population being nursed in that particular ward.

Table 3 shows the length of stay of the case study children. Of course, the children who were observed for 4 days may not have been discharged then, but may have stayed for a further period of time.

The evidence from the ward sister studies appeared to support the notion that the patient allocation ward was substantially busier than the task allocation ward, particularly in terms of the number of interactions in which each sister engaged. The patient allocation sister was observed to engage in a total of 942 interactions (self-initiated and other-initiated) over the 3-day period, while the task allocation sister engaged in a total of 651 interactions. These data also offer clues as to how the task allocation sister perceived and

Table 3 Number of days individual children were observed

No. of days observed	No. of children	
	PA	TA
1	0	0
2	2	1
3	3	1
4	7	9

PA = patient allocation, TA = task allocation

performed her work in terms of social activity, because it was clear that, although she had potentially more time to spare over and above the clinical and administrative demands of the ward and the patients, she chose to spend this time engaged in non-sociable activities, e.g. reading notes, writing lists, up-dating records, etc. (there were 45 recorded instances of non-social activities for one day). Even when the sister engaged in a non-social activity that had potential for social interaction, she did not exploit it:

> 'Sister Albut (*the names of the staff and patients have been changed in order to maintain anonymity*) looks at the diabetic charts on Azia's bed, and she takes Jimmy off a 4-hourly chart and looks at Farah's chart.'

This quoted instance took place in a four-bedded area where children were situated, but the sister ignored them. On the first morning of the study the sister was observed sitting at her desk from 10.20 hrs to 11.40 hrs, during which time she had a cup of tea, talked to the junior sister, did the off-duty, talked to a sales representative, answered the phone and talked to the researcher. At times a child could be heard crying on the ward. The patient allocation sister was noted to be engaging in non-social activity on 23 occasions over a period of 1 day.

On closer examination, it was noted that some of these activities were directly related to 'people comfort', e.g. making tea and toast for a mother. Even when she was engaged in primarily non-social activity, she often used the opportunities for social interaction:

> 'Sister admires Jackie's special cup, which has a straw-like structure down the side ... she looks at Norris's maths problems; they are Fletcher maths.'

The task allocation sister, in contrast, concerned herself primarily with objects to do with the administration of the ward, e.g. paperwork.

This initial impression of the two sisters, taken in the context of the two different ward environments, would lead one to believe that the patient allocation sister was more concerned with the human population of her ward, while the task allocation sister appeared to focus on the jobs that the ward generated, e.g. moving beds, writing labels and requisitions, and liaising with dietitians and engineers. That is not to say that these areas of work were unimportant, but it would appear that these matters took precedence. She concerned herself very little with direct contact with the children and their families:

> 'Sister Albut then goes around the patients with the kardex in her hand. She says "Hello" to John and looks at the little black box on his back (*for monitoring fits*) . . . She says "Hello" to Alwyn's mother . . . She looks at Haji's buttocks and asks the researcher to take a look. She looks at Angela, and asks the nurse if she has got the plastic drawsheet single. She says, "It doesn't need to be double".'

> 'Sister Albut goes to check whether the diabetic urines have been tested and she looks at the charts. She passes the new patient's visitors on the way but she doesn't speak to them.'

Both sisters were asked to give some information about their own personal biographies.

The patient allocation sister was in her mid-30s with a good general educational background (up to 'A' level standard). Her professional qualifications were appropriate to her practice area, and she had engaged in some advanced study to Diploma level. Her work experience had been varied, e.g. work abroad, geriatrics, work as a waitress. She had been on the patient allocation ward for 7 years, and had also worked as a staff nurse with the task allocation sister on the task allocation ward for 2 years.

The task allocation sister was in her early 40s. She had continued her education up to 'O' level standard. She, too, was appropriately qualified for her area of practice, but she had not engaged in any advanced study. Her work experience was, likewise, varied, e.g. agency work, work abroad, rheumatology and work with premature babies. She had been the sister on the task allocation ward for 14 years.

It would appear that the patient allocation sister fits Pembrey's (1978) model more closely, since her educational qualifications were good and she had progressed her professional qualifications to an advanced level.

WORK ROLE PERCEPTIONS AND PRIORITIES

Both sisters were asked how they saw their work roles, and defined their work priorities.

The patient allocation sister said that her prime responsibility was for the patient's welfare, and that she saw the patient as part of the family unit. She went on to include the supervision and teaching of learners, working with the doctors and generally acting as a liaison/mediator between the patient and the rest of the hospital staff. She expressed her responsibility for teaching the junior trained staff on her ward, and for maintaining the principles of the Health and Safety at Work Act. In response to a question about work priorities, she said that the most important ones to her were interaction with the family unit, teaching nurses in order to ensure good standards and creating a happy working atmosphere.

The task allocation sister saw her work role in very different terms. She mentioned being responsible for the organisation of the ward, and for ensuring that the learners got satisfactory experience and adequate supervision, and also saw communicating with parents, other staff and patients (in that order) as part of her job.

She was unable to define priorities – 'Everything is important' – but, when pressed to suggest work that she could leave out, she mentioned serving meals, bedmaking, the afternoon writing of the care list and medicine rounds. This was worrying because it was in these activities that the sister spent a great deal of her time. It would have been interesting to have pursued this further, by asking what she would have done with her time were these activities to be totally delegated. In a crude analysis of the work list (which the sister used daily for the designation of tasks) during the week of the ward sister study, she had been listed on two occasions for bedmaking, two occasions for medicines and one occasion for medical rounds.

WORK ROLES IN REALITY

During the ward sister study it was possible to confirm these statements of commitment to a large extent.

Patient allocation sister

Out of a total of 585 patient allocation sister-initiated interactions, 26% were with the children, 11% with visitors and 2% with both (figure 8). The task allocation sister initiated interactions on a total of 382 occasions, of which 19% were with the children, 14% with visitors and 1% with both (figure 8).

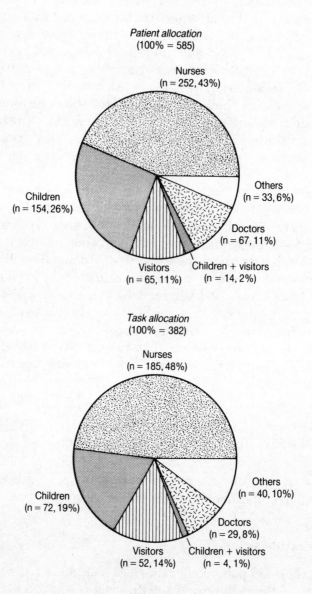

Patient allocation
(100% = 585)

Nurses
(n = 252, 43%)

Children
(n = 154, 26%)

Others
(n = 33, 6%)

Doctors
(n = 67, 11%)

Visitors
(n = 65, 11%)

Children + visitors
(n = 14, 2%)

Task allocation
(100% = 382)

Nurses
(n = 185, 48%)

Children
(n = 72, 19%)

Others
(n = 40, 10%)

Doctors
(n = 29, 8%)

Visitors
(n = 52, 14%)

Children + visitors
(n = 4, 1%)

Figure 8 Interactions initiated by sisters with others

King et al (1971) make the point that the heads of child-oriented units interacted more frequently and more warmly with the children than did the heads of institutionally oriented units.

It has already been argued that the increased rate of interaction by the patient allocation sister could be due, to some extent, to functional reasons, i.e. the 'busy-ness' of the ward. However, on closer examination of the data, it was found that not only were the interactions quantitatively greater, but that the interaction content was of a warmer, less superficial nature:

'Sister assists the nurses with Jackie, who is having a little difficulty with her drugs. She says, "That's a good girl". The child is on her mother's lap being dried after having a bath. "You can have some cucumber sandwiches with the crusts cut off," says Sister. The phone rings. Sister says to Amrit, "Answer the phone then, Doc". Amrit, who is 13, is sitting at the desk with a stethoscope round his neck . . . She tells Amrit that he is like all the other doctors because she is having to fill in all the forms for them. She says, "Have you listened to his chest?" (indicating another child). "Yes," he says, "it's a bit bad." "Does he need any medicine?", asks Sister. She checks Amrit's drugs while hanging onto the phone. Amrit pinches a sterile syringe off the trolley – no-one minds. He pretends to give the other boy an injection. He asks the boy to pretend to start to cry . . . Another Asian boy comes and asks for a syringe. Sister says, "Yes, if you take one while I'm not looking." "Why?", asks the child. "Because it's against the hospital rules," says Sister, "so if you take one when I'm not looking, I won't see, will I?" "Yes," says the child, and takes a syringe.'

The above style of interaction was never witnessed in relation to the task allocation sister. There was no blurring of the boundaries between the sister and the children. Children were not encouraged to play with medical equipment, nor allowed to venture into areas of the ward associated with staff work, e.g. the kitchen or the treatment room. Opportunities for sociable interaction were either not exploited at all or were minimally exploited, as in the example below.

'Edwin (who is five) has lost five pence in the Mickey Mouse phone; Sister asks him whom he is ringing up. "His Nan," says another boy. Edwin says, "It's not ringing." Sister presses the phone and says, "Have you got a dialling tone now?" "Yes," says Edwin and carries on dialling. Sister looks at the fluid balance charts on the desk. Edwin says, "Now!" to the other boy, who is in charge of inserting the money, but he can't get it in and messes it up, so Edwin has to try again and again. Sister says to him, "I don't think you know what you're doing . . ." Edwin gives the researcher the phone to listen to – there is an engaged tone, and I tell him this. Sister says, "Put it down and try later." The boys move away looking crestfallen. Sister puts an antiseptic spray in the treatment room and reads the work list. She checks the specimen bottle drawer.'

This was one of the task allocation sister's longer interactions with the children; most of her sociable interactions with the patients consisted of just saying, "Hello".

The numbers of interactions for sociable reasons initiated with the family units by each of the sisters is illustrated in table 4. In numerical terms, the difference between the two sisters' initiated sociable interactions was considerable, e.g. patient allocation sister = 70, task allocation sister = 18. This was also reflected in the child-initiated interactions: patient allocation sister = 16, task

Table 4 Sociable interactions initiated by the sisters and the children and their visitors

	Sister-initiated interactions				Children/visitor-initiated interactions			
	Patient allocation		Task allocation		Patient allocation		Task allocation	
	n	%	n	%	n	%	n	%
With children	70	79	18	62	16	84	4	67
With visitors	14	16	9	31	3	16	2	33
With both	5	6	2	7	–	–	–	–
Total	89[1]	100	29[2]	100	19[3]	100	6[4]	100

1. 38% of total patient allocation sister-initiated interactions with child/visitors (n = 233)

2. 23% of total task allocation sister-initiated interactions with child/visitors (n = 128)

3. 18% of total patient allocation child/visitor–initiated interactions (n = 104)

4. 17% of total task allocation child/visitor–initiated interactions (n = 35)

N.B. Figures 0.5 and above have been rounded up; those below 0.5 have been rounded down.

allocation sister = 4. The level of sociable interaction between the patient allocation sister and the children is four times greater than the task allocation sister's sociable interactions.

It would seem from the evidence thus far that the patient allocation sister's claim to be concerned with the patients was substantiated. There was more evidence relating to this in the nature of the verbal ward reports, but this will be discussed more fully in the section dealing with work organisation.

The second area of work mentioned by the patient allocation sister in relation to her role was that of supervisor and teacher of learners. Although it was not possible to isolate this area of work from the interaction table, it was, nevertheless, observed to take place on several occasions:

> 'Nurse Duveen comes into the office and discusses her drug assessment, which is to take place later today. Sister Bottomly takes out the assessment forms from the desk and runs through them with her, pointing out the areas where failure is certain if mistakes are made and areas where mistakes are not crucial. She asks the nurse if she would like to hang on to a copy of the form to look at later. The nurse takes a copy away.'

The sister later arranged for Nurse Duveen to have a trial run in readiness for her drug assessment. She was also observed orientating a nurse new to the ward. The verbal ward reports were used for teaching purposes, and also as opportunities for exchanging information, as were the routine drug rounds.

Over the 3-day observation period, the patient allocation sister interacted on 125 occasions with the learners – this accounted for 21% of the sister's total interactions and 50% of the sister's interactions with nursing staff alone (table 5).

On the other hand, the learners initiated interactions on 38 occasions with the sister (table 5; see also figure 9). This constituted 11% of the total number of interactions initiated by 'others' and 30% of the interactions solely initiated by nursing staff. This low number of interactions initiated by the learners (compared with 73 on the task allocation ward) could be explained in various ways:

- that the learners were afraid to initiate interactions with the sister;
- that the ward was not busy enough to warrant more interaction;

Table 5 Interactions by sisters and nurses according to nurse grade

	Sister-initiated interactions				Nurse-initiated interactions			
	Patient allocation		Task allocation		Patient allocation		Task allocation	
	n	%	n	%	n	%	n	%
Auxiliaries	16	6	19	10	6	5	9	6
Learners	125	50	99	54	38	30	73	48
Trained	82	33	53	29	83	65	70	46
*Mixed group	29	12	14	8				
Total	252[1]	100	185[2]	100	127[3]	100	152[4]	100

1. 43% of total patient allocation sister-initiated interactions (n = 585)
2. 48% of total task allocation sister-initiated interactions (n = 382)
3. 36% of total patient allocation other-initiated interactions (n = 357)
4. 57% of total task allocation other-initiated interactions (n = 269)

* The sisters are able to interact with the staff collectively.

N.B. Figures 0.5 and above have been rounded up; those below 0.5 have been rounded down.

● that the learners had enough information, were sufficiently confident for the competent undertaking of their work and could, therefore, operate more autonomously.

The data tend to support the latter theory, particularly in the area of the admission of the sick child, which will be discussed in chapter 4. By implication, this tends to suggest that the patient allocation sister was successful in her work role in relation to learner supervision and teaching.

The evidence to support the role of the patient allocation sister as a liaisor tended to be found in the interactions of the sister with others. On the whole, this involved the sister negotiating with medical staff in the arena of technical care for patients (table 6). However, the category of 'other staff' also included anyone working in the hospital, e.g. domestics, porters, pharmacists, school teachers, physiotherapists, etc., with whom the sister needed to negotiate on the patient's behalf, and on whose services she relied to provide the appropriate environment and facilities for

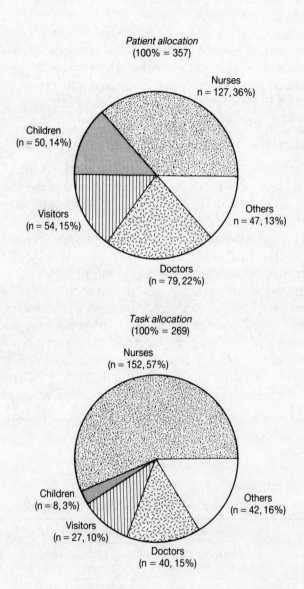

Figure 9 Interactions initiated by others with sisters

patient care, e.g. clean linen, adequate drugs and well-maintained equipment. Taken overall, the patient allocation sister initiated interaction with, and responded to interaction initiated by, others on a total of 226 occasions.

On the whole, the patient allocation sister and her staff took into account individual patient preferences and needs when engaging in negotiations on the patient's behalf. For instance, during a report session, the junior sister discussed the arrangements for taking a child to another hospital for treatment:

> 'He's going to S— hospital today in an old-fashioned taxi – because there is more room for him, his mum, the nurse and the equipment.'

The patient allocation sister initiated interaction with doctors on 67 occasions (see table 6); these constituted 11% of the total patient allocation sister-initiated interactions. Forty (60%) of these interactions were for technical reasons, e.g. the sister asked a doctor to change a prescription. This would appear to support the assumption that technical routines are imposed by the medical staff. Extra support for this assumption might be found in the level of doctor-initiated interactions, which numbered 79 (22%) of total 'other-' initiated interactions, of which 48 (61% doctor-initiated interactions) were for technical reasons. Previous sociological writings have asserted that the doctors' power and control in the arena of patient treatment and the nurses' role in the delivery of that treatment is considerable. Fretwell (1978, p.327) notes the functions of nurses as agents for absent doctors who can be:

> 'confident that a disciplined workforce will carry out their orders and do the work they do not want to do.'

Table 6 Interactions between sisters and non-nursing staff

	Sister-initiated interactions				Other-initiated interactions			
	Patient allocation		Task allocation		Patient allocation		Task allocation	
	n	%	n	%	n	%	n	%
Doctors	67	67	29	42	79	63	40	49
Other staff	33	33	40	58	47	37	42	51
Total	100	100	69	100	126	100	82	100

However, on closer examination of the transcript, it appeared that the patient allocation sister was exhibiting covert control over the work of the doctors and was engaging in considerable negotiation as to what they were allowed to do on the ward in terms of treating and managing the patient flow. The previously quoted example of the sister asking a doctor to change a prescription became more elaborate, as the doctor fetched the prescription sheet and changed it under the sister's watchful eye. The direction of control may seem more understandable and possibly inevitable, in view of the fact that the doctor was very junior and the sister was very experienced (both actors were women). However, a later incident revealed something of the sister's relationship with more senior doctors, when a female consultant arrived on the ward and the sister grumbled about patients arriving on the ward unannounced from the clinic. The consultant looked sheepish and apologised.

The evidence thus far discussed would appear to suggest that there is considerable congruity between how the patient allocation sister conceptualised and actually practised her work role.

Task allocation sister

In the interview, the task allocation sister saw her work as being concerned with ward organisation, providing satisfactory learner experience and supervision and maintaining good communication with parents.

Although the sister did not elaborate on this in the interview, it seemed, from the observation of her practice, that the ward organisation took the form of duties connected with ward administration and housekeeping, as distinct from the organisation of the nurses' work, which will be discussed later.

It will be recollected that the ward administration/housekeeping interaction category concerned anything related to the organisation or management of the ward and the maintenance of a hygienic/safe environment. Table 7 shows the frequency of both sisters' interactions with nurses and others for administrative/housekeeping purposes. In proportional terms, the task allocation sister initiated interaction for administrative purposes slightly more often than did the patient allocation sister (25% of all initiated interaction, compared to 23%). However, it is the amount of interaction initiated by others in this category that is more striking (38% on the task allocation ward and 22% on the patient allocation ward).

Table 7 Interactions initiated by sisters and others in relation to ward administration and housekeeping

	Sister-initiated interactions				Other-initiated interactions			
	Patient allocation		Task allocation		Patient allocation		Task allocation	
	n	%	n	%	n	%	n	%
Nurses	87	64	61	63	42	53	64	63
Children/ visitors	22	16	10	10	9	11	3	3
Non-nursing staff	27	20	26	27	28	35	34	34
Total	136[1]	100	97[2]	100	79[3]	100	101[4]	100

1. 23% of total patient allocation sister-initiated interactions (n = 585)
2. 25% of total task allocation sister-initiated interactions (n = 382)
3. 22% of total patient allocation other-initiated interactions (n = 357)
4. 38% of total task allocation other-initiated interactions (n = 269)

N.B. Figures 0.5 and above have been rounded up; those below 0.5 have been rounded down.

There were several examples in the task allocation sister study that demonstrated the task allocation sister's preference for 'object' rather than 'people' work, and for promoting that preference in others:

> 'Sister asks Nurse Grant, who is holding Alison's (a Downs' Syndrome toddler) breakfast, to clean the suction apparatus at Alison's bedside.'

> 'An Asian girl asks Sister for the toilet. "Look, there's a nurse down there," says the sister pointing.'

In the interview, the task allocation sister stated that there was often a lull on the ward before lunchtime, and one of the alternatives for filling this time was to use it for teaching purposes. During the 3-day sister study, she was not observed actively engaging in teaching, nor was teaching observed to occur during the child studies.

When the sister discussed how she delegated the work, she said that the auxiliaries were usually given the chronically sick children, who were considered to be 'heavy' patients, requiring frequent 'basic' care and being unlikely to recover. However, if the ward was not too busy, the learner nurses were sometimes allowed to care for these patients because the sister felt it was 'good experience' for them:

> ' . . . but even these "heavy" patients may be given to several staff in a day because of the strain of looking after them, the frustrations of feeding, etc.'

This gave some insight into the perceptions of the task allocation sister regarding certain patients. It appeared that she saw the more technically interesting patients as being more relevant for the educational needs of the learners, that these were the patients that generated 'busy-ness' and that the chronically ill with poor prognoses could, on the whole, be cared for by untrained auxiliary help.

As has already been mentioned on the first observation day, in the lull before lunch, the task allocation sister remained in her office from 10.05 hrs to 11.40 hrs, during which time she made a notice for the front of the desk diary, which instructed the staff that only the sisters and the ward clerk could enter forthcoming admissions in the diary and that the information must include age, name, diagnosis and designated consultant. She complained to the junior sister about the nurses not writing in the diary properly. She left the office at 11.45 hrs when a new admission arrived. In the later discussion of the children's admission experience, it was noted that the sister took very little interest in these events. However, on this occasion, she did greet the family and took part in the siting of the patient's bed. This could be explained by the fact that the child was a frequent in-patient to the ward and was going to be treated soon after admission with a plasma infusion. The sister had stated in the interview that she got satisfaction from patients whom she knew well, about whom she could teach the nurses. She was not, however, observed in overt teaching activities involving long-term patients – or any other category of patient for that matter.

It would seem, therefore, that the task allocation sister saw learner experience and supervision purely in terms of organising the work, and not as a direct interactional activity on her part with the learners. Figures 10 and 11 show the interactional level between both sisters and the learners.

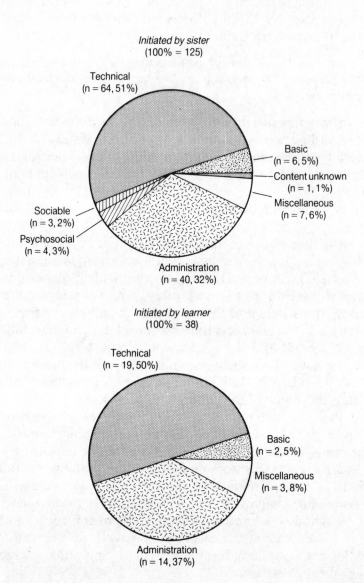

Figure 10 Interactions between patient allocation sister and learners

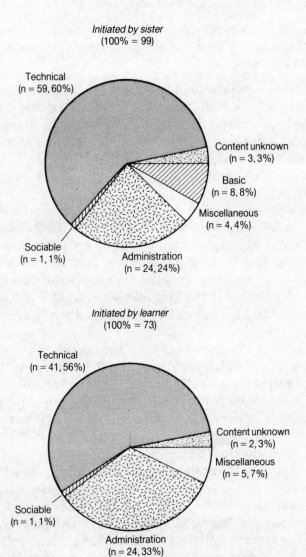

Figure 11 Interactions between task allocation sisters and learner

The task allocation sister mentioned communication as part of her work role; she obviously saw this as an area of significance because later in the interview, when asked about topics of importance, she again mentioned it:

'The consultant sees parents before consulting me and is often not up to date. There are too many people around and you must be careful about communication.'

These comments appear to indicate that the task allocation sister felt some threat to her control of the situation from the 'uncontrolled' communication by the doctors with the parents. Her concern appeared to be that there was too much communication by 'others', rather than that her own role and contribution in the communication process might be deficient or more effective.

On a quantitative basis, the task allocation sister initiated interaction on 382 occasions with 'others' over the 3-day period, while the patient allocation sister interacted on 585 occasions (see figures 8 and 9). It would seem, therefore, that the task allocation sister actually communicated less than the patient allocation sister. It could be argued that as the task allocation ward was less busy, it was not necessary for the task allocation sister to communicate as much.

There were also differences between the two wards concerning the quality of the verbal reports, which will be discussed later. A large proportion of the task allocation sister's communication was achieved via routines, notices and lists. As patients and parents were individuals, their individual needs often fell outside the remit of these strategies, which then became ineffectual in addressing the individual dimensions of care.

Figure 9 (see above) indicates that 152 (57%) of all other-initiated interactions were by nurses. Table 5 (above) shows how these are distributed according to the nurses' grades.

It will be noted that the nurses needed to initiate interaction on a total of 152 occasions with the task allocation sister. It will also be seen, from table 7, that more than a third of these interactions (64) were for reasons of administration. Parents and children, on the other hand, initiated interaction on only 35 occasions (see table 4). The reason for this is open to speculation and not immediately apparent. However, it has already been noted that this sister spent a large proportion of her time in her office attending to administrative matters and, perhaps, when individuals, i.e. parents of sick children, are in a vulnerable position, it takes a great deal of courage and a well-integrated personality to knock on an office door to seek information.

The dimension of staff-initiated interaction on the task allocation ward was rather different from that on the patient allocation ward, inasmuch as the task allocation nurses initiated interaction on a greater number of occasions (152 compared to 127, see figure 9). The reasons for the lower number of nurse-initiated interactions on the patient allocation ward was discussed earlier, but it is also important to consider possible reasons for the higher frequency of nurse-initiated interaction on the task allocation ward. One explanation could be that the task allocation nurses had insufficient information on which to base their nursing actions and needed to refer more to the nurse in charge.

There was also an intriguing phenomenon that was reminiscent of the Tower of London, in that it involved the almost ceremonious handling of the drug cupboard keys by the task allocation sister and the ward staff. The keys to the controlled drugs cupboard are traditionally kept on the person of the nurse in charge of the ward; in practice any nurse whose name appears on a statutory register may check and/or administer such drugs (the procedural details of this are usually determined by local institutional policies). In a ward setting where a number of registered nurses are working together, albeit in a hierarchical situation, there is movement of the controlled drug cupboard keys between them. However, it became clear from observation of the task allocation ward sister that she maintained the tradition of holding the keys, which became an instrument of her control over the activities of the staff, who were required to request the keys and inform her of why they needed them. The control of the keys had wider implications than simply the management of the controlled drugs, because other keys to other medication cupboards were an integral part of the bunch.

'A nurse comes for the keys. Sister Albut says, "What do you want them for?" "Inhalations", says the nurse. She is given the keys and goes.'

By way of contrast, it has already been noted that the patient allocation sister was approached on 127 occasions by the nurses (see figure 9), which, considering the extra 'busy-ness' factors of the patient allocation ward, was considerably less frequent than on the task allocation ward (152 occasions). The phenomenon of the keys was not apparent. This could indicate a greater diversification of power and control and the facilitation of greater personal initiative on the part of the nursing staff.

There was more interaction initiated by the children and parents with the patient allocation sister; this amounted to 104 occasions (29% of all 'other-' initiated interactions). On the task allocation ward, parents and children initiated contact on only 35 occasions (13% of all 'other-' initiated interactions) (see figure 9). This could indicate the increased availability of the patient allocation sister for communication with family units, and the willingness of the families to interact with her. The *Which?* (Consumers' Association, 1985) article emphasised that:

'Parents also need to be given information by knowledgeable and expert staff.'

The willingness and communication competence of trained nurses would seem to be crucial to the two-way flow of information between the ward and the family unit.

Work priorities

The patient allocation sister maintained that her work priorities were interaction with the children and their parents, teaching learners (which helped to maintain a high standard of care) and creating a happy working environment. The ward sister study tended to support these assertions. The sister's interactions with the parents and children were of a high standard as regards both quantity and quality, as has already been discussed in the section on work role. The teaching of learners has also been addressed. There would appear to be some consistency in how the sister sees her work role and the reflection of this in her work priorities.

The atmosphere on the ward was one of flexibility; this was manifested by nurses playing with the children during work as well as when work schedules had been completed. The trained staff were able to meet informally and socially with out-patient families at the Tuesday coffee mornings that were a special feature of the patient allocation ward. This involved making a room available for families visiting the out-patients department. Coffee, squash and biscuits were provided, and the families came and went as they wished. They were usually joined by the nurses at some point, and occasionally parents of in-patients would join in too.

The ward cared for children suffering from malignant and often fatal diseases. This generated a great deal of anxiety among the staff. The sister acknowledged this by attempting to implement a staff support group. This, however, foundered due to the conflict regarding the aims of the group. This was generated by the non-nurses who were there by invitation only; for instance, the doctors wanted to use the sessions to teach the nurses about cancer in children, and the medical social worker wanted to use the time for case conferences.

The patient allocation sister was also observed introducing and familiarising a new nurse with the ward geography and the work organisation philosophy. She showed awareness of situations that generated anxiety and was prepared to take action to reduce this. The use of space for living-in mothers has already been discussed, but it is another example of her concern for the social climate in which the population of the ward, both lay and professional, existed.

The task allocation sister found work priorities difficult to define. She believed that everything was important. When pressed to state what she would be happy to leave out, she mentioned bedmaking, meals, drug rounds and writing lists. Evidence yielded by the work lists for the week in which the ward sister study was carried out shows that this sister was listed on two occasions for bedmaking and on two for drug rounds.

It was interesting that three out of four of the items that she mentioned were those that would ultimately bring her into contact with the patients and their relatives. She did not appear to see work priorities in terms of people, but in terms of the tasks to be carried out.

Although the sister was listed for certain jobs on the work list, an examination of the task allocation sister study transcript showed that, over the 3-day period, she was engaged in bedmaking only once; she was not observed at all in the serving of meals; she was seen to engage in the administration of drugs on six occasions, but only one of these was a 'full blown' drug round. She was, however, observed writing lists, notices and labels on 14 occasions. This evidence would seem to support the notion that the task allocation sister's work preference was for activities that were not directly people-centred. This was quantitatively demonstrated by the total number of interactions initiated by the two sisters. The patient allocation sister initiated interactions on 585 occasions over 3 days, while the task allocation sister initiated interactions on 382 occasions for a similar time span (see figure 8).

CONSTRAINTS IN RUNNING THE WARD

During the interviews, both sisters were asked what constraints prevented them from running the ward the way they would like to. They each perceived these very differently in terms of role creation and role constraints.

The patient allocation sister: role creation

The patient allocation sister saw her own deficiencies as a manager as one of the major constraints on running the ward as she would like to. This could be taken as an indication that the patient allocation sister was acknowledging her ability to create her own role, rather than having it imposed upon her by others; nevertheless, she was able to highlight some of the difficulties encountered in role creation, e.g. maintaining motivation, lack of time, etc., which could, of course, be due to external constraints, such as poor administrative support, failure to acknowledge what she was trying to achieve and demands on her time in terms of paperwork for bureaucratic purposes.

She also mentioned certain elements of environmental determinism, in terms of the geographical layout of the ward, which did not lend itself to coping with the needs of the public, particularly visiting parents, e.g. because of lack of space. However, the sister was able to overcome this to some extent by her own innovation. She was observed, during the sister study, making alternative arrangements for parents when the official accommodation was not available, e.g. mothers were 'put up' in armchairs, empty beds and camp beds in the coffee room.

In terms of other external constraints, the patient allocation sister mentioned the unreliability of the maintenance staff and the unpredictability of the doctors' rounds. These two areas were not noted as problems during the sister study, but it is possible that the nature of the data collection did not expose these areas of concern – doctors' rounds came and went, and it was not possible to establish whether they occurred when expected, nor were overt comments regarding the doctors' unpunctuality noted. The researcher's own ward sister experiences suggest that problems with doctors' rounds centred around the unco-ordinated nature of the visits of junior and senior medical staff, which demanded the presence of a trained nurse, regardless of the doctors' seniority. Similarly, problems with maintenance were found to be infrequent, but, when they did occur, they were so irritating and disruptive as to increase their memorability.

Task allocation sister: role constraints

The task allocation sister viewed constraints solely in terms of things external to herself; she did not demonstrate, in the interview, any acknowledgement of her own role creativity.

The constraints mentioned by the task allocation sister included the implementation of the Health and Safety at Work Act, e.g. having to move collection points for specimens from the main corridor to the sluice, although the original collection point was conveniently situated just outside the sister's office, and, although she did not actually state this, it was implied that the sluice was not very convenient. Perhaps the fact that she had to pass through the patient area to get to the new placement may have been of relevance.

The task allocation sister was also irritated at having the nursing process imposed on her by the nursing hierarchy. The unpunctuality of the consultant ward rounds also occasioned comment. These constraints appeared to affect only the activities of the sister. She did not mention the effect of external constraints on the welfare of the patients and their families. When discussing the effect of constraints on running the ward, perhaps it should have been important to establish for whom or for what one was running the ward – for the benefit/convenience of patients, of staff or even of both.

WORK ORGANISATION

To establish the style of work organisation on each of the wards, the interview discussions focused on what the sisters saw as a 'typical' day and the way in which the nurses were actually deployed in order to complete the work.

The patient allocation sister

The patient allocation sister discussed the work organisation from her own viewpoint, although she acknowledged the fact that there was a patients' point of view. She implied that the work organisation flowed from the needs of the patients:

> 'I rush up to the ward about 10 minutes early and have a quick run around the patients to assess their dependency, before I have a report from the night staff and later go and have a closer look at the patients.'

The nurses were organised on a patient allocation team system. This was done on the basis of the sister's own observations of the patients and of what she learned from the night report. A junior and senior nurse were allocated together to care for half of the ward, with a 'runner' (extra nurse) helping between the two teams. She endeavoured to keep the same nurses allocated to a particular section of the ward for at least a week, but if staff movement was inevitable, she tended to move the trained staff. The teams sorted out the allocation of the individual patients democratically. This system of work organisation had altered slightly since the completion of the data collection, when the sister had allocated the nurses to individual patients herself. She had initiated the change because she found previously, when counselling the junior learners, that they had felt they were not getting enough supervision and were afraid to be left alone with patients.

This change of work organisation by the sister, as a result of the opinions of the junior staff, indicated a willingness both to listen to those less qualified and to change in the light of those opinions. This could also be taken as substantial evidence to support the idea that the patient allocation sister was a democratic leader who was concerned about staff morale and the quality of patient care.

The patient allocation sister used both staff and patient routines as reference points for work organisation, e.g. patients' lunches, report sessions, doctors' rounds, etc.

The sister study confirms most of the statements that the sister made about work organisation. The only area of non-confirmation concerned that of the slightly modified allocation system, as this was introduced following the completion of the sister study. However, it was possible to confirm this during the final child study, as this was carried out after the change had been made.

The problems associated with the possibility of idealising a 'typical day' are acknowledged. However, it became clear from the sister study that the patient allocation sister's description of a 'typical day' on her ward was a fairly accurate reflection of what went on as observed in the ward sister study. Events, of course, do not occur in the neat and tidy way of an interview narrative, e.g. on day 3 of the sister study, the patient allocation sister had accompanied four sets of doctors on rounds before 10.30 a.m. The sister was able, nonetheless, to exploit this situation for interaction with children, parents and staff for a variety of reasons. For example, she asked a group of children to try to blow an ophthalmoscope light out, answered a teacher's query about a child going to school, instructed a learner about arresting a nose bleed, invited a staff nurse to join the round so that she could obtain some information about a patient that she required, gave a child some analgesia and showed a visitor where a child's cot was. She was continuously aware of the world around her and interacted fully with it.

The patient allocation sister saw a 'typical day' in very broad terms of specific activities. Although she mentioned the round of the patients to assess dependency, she was observed in the 3-day study to engage in a considerable amount of high quality interaction with children, which acknowledged them as social beings with individual characteristics, e.g. 233 of the total sister-initiated interactions (585) were with children and visitors, of which 70 were with children for sociable reasons (see table 4).

Although the sister mentioned a specific time of day for talking to parents, she was observed engaging in this activity continuously; 11% (65) of the sister's initiated interactions were with visitors (see figure 8).

Task allocation sister

The task allocation sister's description of a typical day did not imply any dilemma as to whether it should be viewed from her own or the patients' perspective. The former perspective was unequivocally offered, and focused on tasks and ward routines, in which the patients' needs seemed to be of secondary importance (parents were never mentioned). The routine appeared to be rigid and very much under the control of the sister. Staff meal breaks were carefully timetabled. The imposition of routines for the staff's/sister's convenience was evidenced by the comment that the toddlers were dressed in their night clothes at 16.00 hrs, before the early shift went off duty. Routine deficit for the patients' benefit was noted when the sister stated that, at 20.00 hrs, the older children could have a drink if they asked!

The task allocation ward sister study tended to confirm the account of the work organisation in the interview. The lack of focus on the patients was reflected in the observations of the sister's initiated interactions with the children, which constituted 19% (72) of the total sister-initiated interactions (382) (see figure 8). Five per cent (18) of the total were for sociable reasons (see table 4). These were of poor quality and often consisted of the sister just saying 'hello'.

In view of the fact that the parents did not figure in the deliberations of the sister in relation to a 'typical day', it was surprising that 14% (52) of the total task allocation sister-initiated interactions were directed at visitors. However, while the percentage is greater than for the patient allocation sister (11%, 65; see figure 8), it should be noted that the task allocation sister interacted less in general and that the quality of the interaction was usually less satisfactory; for example:

> 'Sister walks down the ward and passes new visitors but doesn't speak to them. She informs Alan's mother about him attending another hospital for treatment and leaves.'

During the doctor's rounds the task allocation sister tended to continue her ward administration activities, e.g. she attended to a notice about stacking the visitors' chairs in the right place, organised treatment for a child with the junior sister, adjusted the work list and asked if a bed was ready for a new admission. She did not engage socially with the child population of the ward.

WORK PRESCRIPTION

Both sisters were asked about how the nurses knew what work they had to do.

Patient allocation sister

The patient allocation sister believed that her management was weak in this area:

'"This is where it falls down", she said.'

She said that the nurses were told about special things happening to their patients and that they were encouraged to ask questions, but never did. The nurses formulated their own care plans under the supervision of the senior nurse, who was in turn supported by the sister. She expected the nurses to think about problems and encouraged them to liaise with the doctors. The nurses also wrote their own kardex reports, and the senior nurses did the lunch-time verbal report.

The patient allocation sister study indicated a high level of good quality communication with the staff. Although the patient allocation sister did not specifically mention the ward report in her discussion of work prescription, she mentioned it several times in her description of a 'typical day' and, by implication, referred to it when she said that the nurses were informed about special things happening to their patients.

Walker (1967), cited in Lelean (1973), identified two functions of the verbal ward report:

1.   to disseminate up-to-date information about the patients, in order for the nurses to care efficiently for them;
2.   to reinforce the social cohesion of the work group by enabling the staff to engage in spontaneous social interaction, which they would not otherwise be able to do because of the nature of their work.

Scales (1958), also in Lelean (1973), defined the functions of the report as:

'(1) to hand over continuation of care of the patients between shifts;
(2) to study the doctors' orders and arrange for them to be carried out;
(3) to implement orders for the ensuing shift.' (p.29)

Perry (1968), on the other hand, saw the function report as follows:

'(1) to comment on patients' condition and progress;
(2) to determine the action to be taken in an emergency;
(3) to report treatments given;
(4) to give instructions for observation and treatment.' (p.29)

Lelean (1973), in her overview of the literature regarding the ward report, discriminated between the written kardex and the verbal report. She maintained that the sisters' main methods of communicating instructions to the nurses were via the written nursing record and the verbal change of shift report. She made no mention of the function of the report for conveying to the staff the nature of patients as individual, social beings. Reports have tended to be regarded as instrumental in nature, without elements of expressiveness. Perhaps further work needs to be done in exploring how powerful reports are in conveying and reproducing attitudes about patients, in relation to patient- and task-centredness.

Lelean (1973) found that written records, while not inaccurate, were often incomplete and ambiguous – the verbal report was seen as a quick way of passing on up-to-date information and encouraging group cohesion. In content, the report was principally about the physical care of the patients, although it could also contain references to the patients' psychosocial needs.

In her conclusion, Lelean suggested that the aim, function and content of both verbal and written reports needed more detailed investigation. She recommended the development of report-giving into patient-centred discussions between members of the ward team, in order to improve standards of care. It was, therefore, decided to analyse verbal reports, as observed in the sister study, in terms of their content, in an attempt to establish whether the ward sister and her staff were patient- or job-orientated. The direction of the interaction during the report might also offer clues as to whether the ward sister was democratic or authoritarian in her leadership style.

During the sister studies, the delivery of the verbal ward reports was observed on a total of 17 occasions (eight on the patient allocation ward and nine on the task allocation ward).

A model of ward report content was constructed, moving along the continuum of patient/task orientation, although it was recognised that, in reality, there could exist elements of different parts of the model encapsulated in the verbal report pertaining to a particular patient (see figure 12).

The final category (6) was difficult to classify, since it could be argued that when patients are no longer medically interesting as disease entities, it is likely that they become marginalised. The use of meaningless expressions, e.g. 'usual day', by the nurse in

1. Individualised basic care according to dependency.
    Appropriate illness-related care, psychosocial support.
    Recognition and acknowledgement of the child and his
    family's individual characteristics and needs. (Nursing
    model of care: patient orientated.)

2. Individualised basic illness-related care, psychosocial
    support and recognition of individual characteristics.

3. Individualised basic and illness-related care.

4. Individualised illness-related care.

5. Illness references only. (Medical model of care: disease
    orientated.)

6. Meaningless, non-quantifiable expressions, e.g. usual day;
    the same; tender, loving care.

Figure 12 Verbal report content

relation to particular patients could indicate that the nurse had
previously perceived these patients in terms of illness features,
and that when these features were no longer amenable to medical
cure (but, nevertheless, still continued to need nursing care), the
status of the patients became eroded and they were barely seen to
exist, even as a work object. (The patient then lies outside, but is,
nonetheless, an extension of, the medical model of care.)

Haralambos (1980) asserts that sociologists must examine the
processes of interaction and endeavour to understand what they
mean and what it is that guides and directs them.

Bearing this in mind, the ward report could prove to be a key
event in terms of explaining how the sister created her role,
functioned as a role model and conceptualised her work. All of
these dimensions could influence whether the patient was treated
as an individual or as a work object.

On the patient allocation ward, the quality of the verbal ward
reports tended towards category 1 of figure 12. In the quantitative

analysis of the ward sisters' activities (see figures 8 and 9), the quality of the reports was obscured, since the report was recorded as one interaction in the technical category (unless the report was interrupted by another initiating interactor). Perhaps a more appropriate method of analysing the ward reports would have been to have dealt with them separately from the main transcript and analysed them in greater detail. However, by examining the transcript closely, it became clear that the patient allocation ward reports were concerned with the children as individuals; not only were the children's present illness state, past medical history and nursing care discussed, but also the children's personal preferences and their psychosocial needs, e.g.:

> 'Stacy ... Age 8, Von Willebrand's Disease – Stacy hasn't liked the taste of her drugs; her parents are divorced and she lives with her father – she seems more settled since these relationships have stabilised.'

The written kardex on the patient allocation ward (which was used as an 'aide memoire' for verbal reports) also contained a list of the individual preferences of the children, e.g. nutritional likes and dislikes. Although no evidence was obtained to confirm how often this record was actually referred to after it had been collected, it appeared to be functional during the admission phase in focusing the attention of the nurse on the child as an individual. The evidence from the child studies also suggested that the care on the patient allocation ward was more individualised, but how much the kardex contributed to this was impossible to determine.

During the patient allocation report sessions there was two-way communication, the sister almost inevitably inviting questions and discussion appearing to flow freely. During one report session, the sister nursed on her knee a sleeping Asian toddler, who subsequently urinated on her during his sleep.

The ward report was a significant event in relation to work prescription – the multidimensional movement of information and the means of reinforcing notions of individuality in terms of the care of the children. However, it was not the only time that there was a dialogue between the sister and the nurses in order for them to know what was going on and, from that, to deduce what to do. Table 5 shows the range of interactions initiated by the sister with all the nurses. It will be noted that the group of nurses with whom she initiated interaction most was the learners. This was a total of 125 (50%) times, of which 64 interactions were for technical reasons and 40 interactions were for administrative reasons (see also table 7).

The evidence in the patient allocation ward sister study transcript showed that the sister was constantly updating the nurses as new information concerning the patients was received by her. This could explain the small number of interactions initiated by the learners (see table 5) – a total of 38 (30%), of which 19 interactions were for technical reasons and 14 for administrative reasons (see also table 7). It is likely that the most rational explanation of this was that the nurses had sufficient information on which to base their nursing actions and needed to refer to the sister only on a limited number of occasions. Perhaps the sister's management of this area was more effective than she at first believed.

Task allocation sister

The task allocation sister mentioned the ward reports, word of mouth, nursing care cards and the nursing care list as the means by which the nurses knew what to do. She also felt that the nurses used their own initiative.

The report sessions on the task allocation ward were very different from those on the patient allocation ward. They tended to focus on the technical needs of the children, along with any administrative issues that required attention. The sister did not engage in two-way discussion – in fact, on the first day of the ward sister study, she did not acknowledge the presence of the assembled staff awaiting the report.

There were occasional references to child distress by other staff (excluding the sister) e.g.:

'Mark, aged 18 months, with asthma – had been pyrexial and his fluids were encouraged; he has been miserable and tearful this morning.'

An interesting feature of the task allocation ward was the number of repeat reports done to cover the same time interval. This was observed at 8 a.m. on the first and third days of the ward sister study. On the first day, the night nurse reported to the assembled day staff, and then left. The day staff nurse then went through the report again, with minor modifications, usually concerning the organisational aspects of the children's care, e.g. the night nurse reported that:

'Matthew, aged 2 years, with cystic fibrosis and chest infection, has slept for long periods, but he is extremely miserable and tearful this morning and looks a bit dusky grey.'

The day staff nurse's repeat account for this child mentioned that he:

'... is for discharge soon, but he is to have a hearing test and he is query for speech therapy because he is rather backward with his speech.'

The day staff left the office after the day staff nurse's version of the report, but the junior sister remained with the task allocation sister (who had just returned from a weekend off) and went through the patients a third time; she commented on Matthew as follows:

'Matthew's mum has been very good with him, and she does his physio four times a day.'

The junior sister offered extra information on most of the children. These extracts from the repeated ward reports illustrate how information was hierarchically organised on the ward. There was sharing of information upwards, but there did not seem to be reciprocal exchange with the more junior staff. The task allocation sister would be extremely well informed and in control as a result of the extra reports, and one questions why the junior sister and staff nurse did not include their information items on the agenda of the night nurse's report in order that knowledge sharing would be equal.

A second good example of the cumulative information gained by the task allocation sister concerned Elizabeth, a 10-year-old, diabetic girl:

'First report   "She's had ketoacidosis and she has got eczema.
(*Night nurse*)   She was a little late to settle.'' Mention was made of
                    her urine results and drug therapy.

Second report   The diabetic treatment is described. ''Her
(*Staff nurse*)   headmaster is coming to see her at 10 a.m. today
                    and she can go to school.''

Third report	"Elizabeth has been very poorly and her parents
(Junior sister)	have not been told about her ketoacidosis, but her

(Junior sister)   father has been giving her portions that have made
her worse. Her parents are going to be taught about
ketoacidosis."

Apart from the hierarchical management of information, it seemed that the junior staff had access to information that related to more immediate matters rather than to more long-term goals. Despite the access to extra information that the task allocation sister had, it did not always facilitate her performance as communicator with the multidisciplinary caring team, e.g.:

'The doctor asked if Angela's diarrhoea had stopped – the sister didn't know, despite its being mentioned three times during the ward report.'

This also posed questions as to what kind of information took precedence in the sister's memory: Angela's diarrhoea was clearly important to Angela, but apparently less so to sister.

It is likely that more efficient use of resources in terms of staffing and time could be made if a more consistent quality of communication and information exchange was achieved. More importantly, it is likely that greater individualisation of care would be facilitated, and support of the child and his/her family improved, if the whole staff had access to all available information, on which they could base their actions.

In addition to the report giving the nurses information about what they should do, the task allocation sister mentioned the nursing care cards, situated at the end of each bed, which stated the nursing care for the individual patient. These had been in use for just 8 days when the interview was carried out. Previously, the same information was recorded in a nursing care list, and the nurses' job allocations were listed underneath the children's names (see figure 13). This latter system was in use during the task allocation sister study.

In the task allocation sister study, there are several examples of the nursing care/task list not functioning, e.g.:

'Sister asks Nurse Rivers if she is looking after Jimmy. "No", says the nurse. "You are," says the sister, "and he hasn't been touched this morning. You'd better go and attend to him."'

Work prescription and allocation on the task allocation ward

Name	Treatment	Bath	P. areas	Oral hygiene	Oral fluids	i.v.	1/O chart	Recordings
Amanda	Physio and School	Big						4-hrly
Richard	Suction PRN	Big			Encourage	✓	✓	
Simon	Liquidised diet	Big					✓	
Kimberley	All nursing care	Bed	2-hrly	2-hrly				
Morning								
9.00 Sister A	Beds. Dr rounds. Medicines							
9.15 SEN	Beds. Nathaniel inhalations							
9.30 N. Marshall	Baths. c/o Christopher and Jeremy							
9.30 N. Lionel	Baths. 4-hrly TPRs John							
9.45 N/A Brown	Baths. c/o Maralyn							
9.45 N/A Rogers	Baths. Drinks, extra fluids							
Coffee break								
Afternoon								
S/N	Medicines							
SEN	c/o Nathaniel							
N. Lionel	c/o Louise and Conrad				All help with			
N. Whitehouse	c/o James & specimens				washes 15.00 hr			
N. Kenny	4-hrly and daily TPRs							
N. Giggetty	c/o Josephine				teas 15.30 hr			
N/A Brown	c/o Maralyn							
N/A Rogers	Drinks and extra fluids – escort John to X-ray							
N. George	c/o Tony							
Evening								
S/N	Medicines. c/o house and James							
N. Whitehouse	c/o Christine and Shahzaz							
N. Giggetty	c/o Tony. 4-hrly TPRs							
N. Kenny	c/o Maralyn							
N. George	c/o toddlers							

Figure 13 Nursing care list (task allocation)

appeared to have changed very little since the data were collected, except for the cards already mentioned. The final child in the task allocation ward child studies was observed after the introduction of the new system. Particular reference will be made to this when examining the child studies.

It is perhaps worth remembering at this point the level of interaction engaged in by the two sisters with the nursing staff on each of the wards. Figure 8 above shows that out of a total of 585 patient allocation sister-initiated interactions, 252 (43%) were with the nursing staff. In contrast, the task allocation sister initiated interaction with her staff 185 (48%) times out of a total of 392 interactions with others. This gives some indication of how the task allocation sister was engaging in less social interaction overall, but it was proportionally greater with the nurses than it was with the patients and families (128 occasions).

On examination of the other-initiated interactions (see figure 9) it will be noted that the nursing staff initiated interaction with the task allocation sister on 152 (57%) occasions out of a total of 269 other-initiated interactions, while, in contrast, the patient allocation ward staff initiated interactions on 127 (36%) occasions out of a total of 357 other-initiated interactions.

An examination of the content of the other-initiated interactions (figure 14), showed that the task allocation nurses interacted almost equally for technical and administrative reasons. This was on 66 (43% of all nurse-initiated interactions)and 64 occasions (42% of all nurse-initiated interactions) respectively. On the other hand, the patient allocation ward staff interacted 61 (48% of all nurse-initiated interaction) times for technical reasons and 42 (33% of all nurse-initiated interaction) times for administrative reasons.

This would appear to support the notion that the task allocation nurses were given little information with which to do their work, particularly in the arena of long-term planning and the organisation of care. While the figures for nurse-initiated interaction for technical and administrative reasons are similar on both wards, they are proportionally larger on the task allocation ward.

PATIENTS' NEEDS

In the interviews, both sisters were asked how the patients' daily and special needs were met.

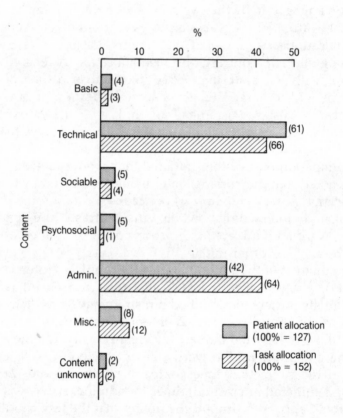

Figure 14   Interaction initiated by nurses on both wards

Patient allocation sister

The patient allocation sister believed that the patients' needs were being met by a system of patient allocation. She felt that the only routines being used to meet patients' needs were meal and drug rounds. This evidence from the ward sister study tended to support the existence of these two routines, and also revealed several others.

It could be argued that patient allocation, which had been changed to a system of team nursing since the collection of the data, is itself a form of work routine. Associated with the patient allocation routine were other routines, such as the use of a special kardex on admission. The sister was sometimes sceptical about how the nurses handled this routine, e.g. when she asked a nurse to show a new colleague how to complete the admission routine doing the nursing process and using a care plan, she added sarcastically:

> '. . . like you've been doing since you've been on the ward.'

The patient allocation sister also had a routine for allocating nurses to patients by writing their names in a book alongside the patient for whom they were responsible. The sister demonstrated annoyance when this system was not adhered to, e.g.:

> 'she has a little bit of an altercation with Sister Duncan about her taking Elspeth's temperature. Elspeth is allocated to one of the nurses. Sister Duncan takes umbrage and says she'll go and sit down out of the way.'

The patient allocation sister, however, was inconsistent on occasions in her own behaviour in relation to allocated children. Later in the sister study she was observed contradicting her patient allocation philosophy by wanting to bath a young child who had been allocated to one of the nurses. This incident was interesting because it was related to a promise she had made to the child about a bath toy:

> 'sister says, "I wanted to do him; oh, all right, you do him, but I promised he could use this toy in the bath." She asks the child if he wants the big bath or the little bath, and he chooses the little bath, so she fixes up the toy on the wall at the side of the bath and shows both of them how it works.'

The sister was also using her authority to introduce the 'pleasure factor' into her work, but was prepared to forego this when the nurse got in first.

There was also evidence in the sister study of routines to do with time and space, which were related to the chronological age of the children, e.g.:

> 'The new patient's mother comes to ask how long they can stay. Staff Nurse Bilson responds with, "Oh, between 7 and 8 o'clock", but sister says, "7 o'clock", and then inquires which part of the ward the child is in. It appears that the child has been admitted into the toddler end of the ward, where they try to put the lights out a little earlier, and, because the mother has confirmed this position, the sister reiterates, "Yes, 7 o'clock." '

The patient allocation sister study confirmed that the sister used a system of patient allocation in order to meet the patients' needs. Evidence of individualised care during the sister study has also been cited, but the question of whether the patients' needs were being met by this system of work organisation will be more fully addressed in the analysis and discussion of the child studies.

Task allocation sister

The patients' needs on the task allocation ward were met mainly by routines. The task allocation sister had modified the organisation of the work marginally since the data collection. This had meant that instead of just having a nursing care list pinned to the wall in the sterile equipment room, the details of this list were replicated (as mentioned earlier) on small cards at the end of each bed, and, while the cards were individualised, the care remained, as before, task allocated. The task allocation sister said that bedmaking, temperatures, specimens and drinks were done routinely.

> 'There is the odd instance where a nurse will "special" a patient and do everything for it.'

The nursing care list (see figure 13, above) (and, of late, the nursing care cards) listed the children's care in terms of basic and technical tasks. The sister often checked the work list, e.g.:

> 'Sister goes to the sterile equipment room and looks at the work list and adjusts it. She talks to the junior sister about a child being saturated up to his neck . . . she looks again at the list and says that the nurse has probably gone to coffee.'

The nursing care list entry for this particular child stated '24-hour EEG, chart fits, oral fluids'.

In the section 'Work prescription – task allocation sister', above, an example of the work list not functioning in relation to Jimmy's care was cited. This same example also shows how the specific work prescription did not always coincide with the patients' care needs, and demonstrated how patients can fall through the net of general work prescription, when the sister implied that the nurse had failed to give Jimmy basic care by saying:

'. . . and he hasn't been touched this morning.'

The specific care prescription for Jimmy on the work list read as follows:

'Observe for breathlessness; weight-reducing diet. Milk only 400 ml daily, and diabetic drinks.'

There was no indication of Jimmy's other needs, except that Nurse Rivers was down on the list to care specifically for Jimmy and another child. Additionally, she was responsible for baths, collecting specimens and 4-hourly temperatures, in general terms, for the whole ward. It was implied in both of these examples that basic care was routine and that the routine formed part of the communication system, i.e. the patient would receive basic care via the non-articulated routines. Precedence in the verbal report and the work list instructions was given to medical aspects of care. Despite the 'non-articulated' routines, both of these patients experienced deficiencies in care, indicating that the routine was not always effective in adequately providing this.

There was no guarantee that the nurses would automatically know what basic care was needed and, if they did know, that they would carry it out. While one of the caveats of patient allocation is the assumption that every nurse is caring, competent and compassionate, a parallel in task allocation is the assumption that the nurse will deliver basic care, when needed, without being told. Implicit in this assumption is a need for a certain degree of autonomy in decision-making and the ability to assess and deliver basic care according to individual needs – qualities not normally associated with task allocation in the professional ideology. The evidence examined thus far would tend to support in part this notion, with some reservations about the centrality of the role of task allocation. Further evidence will be presented to support this view in the chapter on the child studies.

The evidence tends to suggest that there was a greater satisfaction of patients' needs on the patient allocation ward, in terms of a more patient-centred approach, which contained a greater degree of sister – patient interaction. It will be demonstrated in the examination of the child studies that this was reflected in the interactions between the patients and the rest of the staff. This suggests that a patient-centred philosophy is more likely to emerge as a result of the type of role model that the ward sister presents. This may be a consequence of her work concepts and practices rather than a result of the pattern of work organisation.

Corwin (1965) notes that:

> 'Because the clients' welfare is not necessarily equivalent to the welfare of the organisation, professional and bureaucratic principles provide competing sources of loyalty. Professional standards are sometimes compromised for efficiency and the organisation's prestige.'

Coser (1963) examined whether:

> 'a routinised mechanical view of tasks and alienation of self in the work situation is associated with a different perception of the social field.'

She found, in her comparative study of nurses working in a rehabilitation unit and of nurses concerned with custodial care, that the patient-orientated nurses (in the rehabilitation unit) had an inclusive view of their work, that is, including the patient as a role partner. This was contrary to Johnson and Martins' later (1965) view that the patient was in no position to assume leadership in the doctor/nurse/patient triad. Perhaps this was an empirical rather than a normative viewpoint, and it appears to be based on multifarious assumptions.

Coser (1963) also found that the patient-orientated nurses saw the ward in terms of the people in it, while the task orientated staff had an exclusive view of their work, in that they described it in restricted terms, i.e. as routine housekeeping tasks. They also perceived themselves as unrelated to others in the work that they did.

The two sisters in the present study would appear to fit these two categories of inclusiveness and exclusiveness in terms of their interactional styles and work conceptualisations. This is further supported by their descriptions of their wards at their most ideal:

'The patient allocation sister was asked how she saw the ward looking at its best. She thought Sunday mornings, when there are no doctors, no odd bods around and the nurses are all back from coffee playing with the kids, there's water, paints and TV, games, a state of quiet play.'

'When the task allocation sister was asked to describe the ward looking at its best, she said facetiously, "When it's empty", but then went on to say, "When everything is running smoothly, and this depends on the age group of the children and whether the parents are sensible or not." She said she had just gone through a nice patch with parents. There had been several sensible ones who respected the nurses and had made nice comments about them.'

These views were reinforced by their descriptions of a typical day, about which the patient allocation sister gave a more people-orientated description, while the task allocation sister focused on the jobs to be done. Their descriptions of a typical day on their wards were reasonably accurate, given the difficulty that most wards are 'unstable' environments in which unpredictability is manifest.

The ward sister studies confirmed this difference in emphasis. The difference in the quantity of sister-initiated interactions was the first clue – patient allocation sister = 585, task allocation sister = 382. The qualitative examination of the data confirmed that the patient allocation sister was patient-centred and the task allocation sister job-centred in the approach to her work.

Fretwell (1978) maintained that the traditional model of nursing was dominated by hierarchy and routine. As a result of a two-stage study (Fretwell, 1978), she suggested that this model contributed to an automatic job performance and inhibited a spirit of enquiry, particularly during routine work.

Coser (1963) has discussed the contribution of automatic job performance as a characteristic of alienation, and Brown (1973) has described the incidence of low intrinsic rewards associated with routine work. Fretwell (1978) goes on to state:

'there was a sense in which a rigid routine ... denuded care of its individuality.'

She believed that this traditional model of nursing has developed from an industrial model and has been adopted as a device to get the work done:

'There is a block prescription of care for different categories of patients, role prescription for staff, so that new and transient staff know what to do, a system of hierarchical task allocation and most important of all, the ward routine.'

Fretwell went on to express concern that the emphasis on rigid routines perpetuated an autocratic style of leadership. This could be facilitated by the form that communication between the ward sister and the staff and patients takes. In this could be invested the sister's own foibles, along with those of the medical staff, and these may be reflected in written instructions and in documentation found in the ward. Indeed, it was observed that there was a proliferation of notices on the task allocation ward.

The first notice recorded in the task allocation ward sister study concerns the stacking of chairs for the use of visitors. This notice had fallen off the wall and the domestic worker was seen holding it – the sister noticed this, asked the domestic for the notice and clipped it to the front of the kardex. Sister was later observed re-sticking the notice carefully to the wall. This notice asked visitors to return their chairs to that particular part of the ward when they had finished with them.

This sister was not only concerned with the notices themselves but also with the means by which they were fixed to surfaces. She was observed removing, from the end of a child's cot, a notice that had been attached with expensive adhesive strapping. She re-applied the notice with sellotape. Later in the observation study she was heard giving a verbal report to the ward staff during which she specifically asked the nurses not to use 'micropore' for sticking on labels.

The task allocation ward sister study described how the sister complained to her junior about the nurses not filling in, in the ward diary, the correct details of in-coming patients. She was observed carefully making a notice for the front of the diary stating:

'Only sisters and the ward clerk are allowed to make entries re expected admissions; the details must include age, name, diagnosis, consultant, etc.'

There were many other notices on the task allocation ward, carrying mainly negative instructions, which were used as a means of control of both staff and public in the sister's absence, e.g. the kitchen door 'No entry to visitors' and staff toilet 'No smoking' notices (both inside and outside). In the sterile equipment room the researcher counted a total of 12 notices.

On the patient allocation ward there were fewer notices, and those that did exist were not the usual official looking instructions but were 'home made' with a 'Mr Men' theme and a rhyme; for example, a nil by mouth notice read:

'You must not eat or drink today,
You've got to have a test,
so Mr Greedy says
"I'll stay – I'll eat your food, that's best."'

If the routine did constitute itself partly in this form of communication, then communication between the sister and the patients and the staff may well have been reduced. Indeed, Fretwell (1978) noted that 'Revans (1964) and Lelean (1973) found that the sister spent less than 1–2% of her time talking to junior nurses'. However, this datum was not supported in the present study, apart from the fact that the patient allocation sister initiated interaction on 585 occasions with all interactors, while the task allocation sister initiated interaction on 382 occasions. However, of these total sister-initiated interactions, just over 20% of the patient allocation sister's were with learners, while the task allocation sister's with learners were 26% of the total. It is, of course, possible that, had the data been analysed using length of time taken by the interactions, rather than the number of interactions, it may have been found that the task allocation sister performed rather less well. The content of her interactions was not of a high quality, e.g. interactions in the category of task allocation sister-initiated sociable interactions with children consisted mainly of the sister saying 'Hello'. Sociable interactions with children by the patient allocation sister were often quite lengthy dialogues.

The question of whether the patients' needs were being met will be discussed more fully in chapter 4 relating to the child studies. However, it would seem, from the evidence discussed in this section, that it is likely that the children's psychosocial needs were not as effectively met as on the patient allocation ward. This could probably be accounted for by the task-centred orientation of the sister, rather than by being a direct result of the method of work organisation.

Accountability

Both sisters in the interview were questioned about how they checked that the nurses had done what they were supposed to have done.

Patient allocation sister

The patient allocation sister mentioned her examination of the charts and the nursing kardex. She also said she observed the patients and asked everyone – nurses, parents, patients or anyone who was around.

The ward sister study tended to confirm that the patient allocation sister used these strategies to extract accountability from her staff. Nurses were observed writing the kardex report on the children they were responsible for; under the new system, the team leader gave a verbal report on his/her group of patients. The ward sister invariably did a round of all the patients, looked at their charts and also used the opportunity to engage in sociable interaction:

> 'Sister says she'll check the charts while she's down here. She notices that it's Surinder's birthday tomorrow. She talks to Vernon's mum and dad. Stacy comes to say "Goodbye". Staff nurse gives sister the keys. Sister asks the girl who's overdosed if she's better and more awake. She asks who is looking after Amrit. It's staff nurse. Sister says, "Wouldn't it be nice to give him a new 4-hourly chart?" Staff Nurse says, "I haven't done his 6 o'clock temperature yet." "Well, someone has", says sister. Staff nurse says, "I don't know who." Sister asks Nurse Northbridge if Elspeth's had a drink since 6 o'clock. "Yes. Ribena." "Well, it's not been charted", says sister.'

Sister was observed several times asking children, staff and parents about treatments and basic nursing care:

> 'Sister asks Alicia if she's had a wash yet. "No," she says. "I'm waiting for my mum to bring my stuff." Her father is there and he says, "That's probably an excuse."'

The patient allocation sister did not rely on records alone to extract accountability, but used her own interactive skills with the population of the ward to find out what was going on.

Task allocation sister

The task allocation sister mentioned similar strategies in her interview. However, during the sister study she appeared to prefer 'paper' to 'people' to maintain accountability, e.g. charts, records, the patient-care list (which the sister referred to as the 'work list'). This was not inconsistent with her approach in other areas of her work. The example of Jimmy has been cited in the discussions on work prescription and patients' needs. The same example also demonstrates how the sister relied on the list for determining accountability.

The task allocation sister also checked the charts, but did not exploit this opportunity to interact with the patients:

'Sister looks at the diabetic charts on Azia's bed, takes Jimmy off his 4-hourly and looks at Farah's chart ... Sister checks Alwyn's charts; she doesn't speak; he's eating his lunch with his mother there.'

On the occasion quoted, many of the children were in the day room eating their lunches, yet the sister did not speak to those who remained behind:

'Sister goes to check whether the diabetic urines have been tested and she looks at the charts. She passes some new visitors on the way, but does not speak to them.'

All of the above quoted instances occurred before lunch on the first observation day. It would seem that the method of extracting accountability could vary according to how the sisters conceptualised their work. There was almost a tendency for the task allocation sister to extract accountability from objects rather than people.

AREAS OF IMPORTANCE TO THE SISTERS

There is no doubt that the ward sister holds a key position in the clinical environment. Pembrey (1980, p.85) stated that:

'the ward sister remains the key nurse in negotiating the care of the patient because she is the only person in the nursing structure who actually and symbolically represents continuity of care to the patient.'

Sisters do, however, experience constraints, frustrations and role conflict in the performance of their work. Both sisters in the study talked about changes in the wards, in learner nurses and in areas of importance in relation to their work.

Patient allocation sister

The patient allocation sister mentioned both negative and positive changes that had taken place on her ward, e.g. extra consultants increasing the work load. The appointment of a haemophilia sister and an oncology staff nurse had helped to counteract this. The patient allocation sister study revealed a high level of medical presence on the patient allocation ward; this will be further examined in the discussion of the child studies. On many occasions, the extra trained staff were observed taking part in the day-to-day activities, and they appeared to be well integrated into the workforce.

The patient allocation sister believed that there were no problems with the learners, that they responded to the way that the ward was run, and that perhaps one in a hundred found it difficult to cope with patient allocation. These tended to be the more senior learners, who, paradoxically, found it difficult to manage the responsibility and needed more supervision and teaching. This insight offered by the patient allocation sister could imply that a task allocation system of work organisation could neutralise excellence and obscure incompetence.

An area of importance to the patient allocation sister was the notion that if patient allocation was more universally practised, the nurses would be more accustomed to it.

Task allocation sister

The task allocation sister mentioned only the negative aspects of ward changes, e.g. the shorter working week (she had previously been used to having the afternoon off; the shorter working week precluded this and she was less able to go on early every day 'to get everything straight'), changes in medical staff, nurses away from the ward longer for study periods, and the coerciveness of the GNC (General Nursing Council, now the United Kingdom Central Council) policy regarding the nursing process. It was not possible to substantiate these points from the data, except to note that the sister came on duty at lunchtime instead of in the early morning. The medical presence was not as great as it was on the patient allocation ward, but this could perhaps be explained by the fact that there were fewer consultants attached to the ward.

The move towards implementing the nursing process was very slight, since the only extra activity carried out was the use of individual cards for each child – the actual work organisation appeared to be unchanged.

PSYCHOSOCIAL SUPPORT

The main area of contrast between the two sisters was in relation to task-/patient-centredness. It was, therefore, important to scrutinise whether a patient-centred approach alerted the patient allocation sister to actual/potential psychosocial distress; if this distress was acknowledged, the way in which it was dealt with would also be significant. Similarly, it was important to establish whether a task-centred approach precluded the acknowledgement and treatment of psychosocial distress by the task allocation sister.

Patient allocation sister

There were no specific questions in the interview schedule aimed at establishing the patient allocation sister's views on the identification and treatment of psychosocial distress. However, she was asked how she saw the ward looking at its best:

'Sunday mornings, when there are no doctors, no odd bods around and the nurses are all back from coffee playing with the kids, there's water, paints and TV, games, a state of quiet play.'

In reply to questions about what was needed on the ward she said:

'A parents' room and a bigger storage space for junk, and a bigger playroom, separate from the dining room because they use the playroom as a dining room; and better play facilities are needed.'

These two responses further support the notion that this sister was patient-centred in her approach to her work. It would seem logical to assume that patient-centredness not only implied a concern for the physical comfort and technological safety of the patients, but that it also included the identification and fulfilment of psychosocial needs.

An examination of the patient allocation ward sister study reveals many examples of the ability of the sister to anticipate and recognise psychosocial distress in both nurses and patients, and to deal with it appropriately:

'A new nurse has come to start work on the ward − sister asks her where she has worked before and if she is enjoying her training ... Sister collects the new nurse from the office and shows her round the ward.'

'Sister assists the nurse with Jackie, who is having difficulty with her drugs. She says, "That's a good girl." The child is on her mother's lap being dried after having a bath. "You can have some cucumber sandwiches with the crusts cut off", says the sister.

'Sister offers a new mother a camp-bed and advises her about supper in the canteen . . . she offers the mother tea and toast . . . asks the mother whether she would like Marmite, marmalade or jam.'

The psychosocial aspects of care are also emphasised in the verbal reports:

'Amrit was fretful at the weekend and tearful at the prospect of an intravenous infusion. He seems better for knowing what's going to happen. His family are trying to get a phone at home. Amrit had a tour around the labs with a white coat on – he was pleased about that.'

'Narib, who is very depressed, took some tablets from her uncle's pocket, plus panadol. She has no apparent problems at home or at school – the drugs were not enough to be dangerous but she has been admitted to find out why she took them. She's quiet and withdrawn – it doesn't help being in a bay with all boys, but there's nowhere else to put her.'

There were sometimes scenes of great pathos, presenting episodes of what would appear to be irremediable distress:

'A child is screaming and begging at the top of the ward. "No lady, please no!" The woman doctor, the haemophiliac sister and his mother hold him down to obtain a blood specimen from a vein. His mother is holding and looking away.'

Nevertheless, the evidence suggested that the patient allocation sister was aware of potential/actual psychosocial distress and, on the whole, that she was able to deal with it appropriately. She also accepted responsibility for the emotional support of her staff and had, as mentioned earlier, attempted to set up a staff support group, which had failed because of conflict of goals with other disciplines, e.g. medical staff and the social worker.

Task allocation sister

Evidence of psychosocial support was difficult to locate. Distress did not appear to be identified and acknowledged as readily as it was on the patient allocation ward. The sister was observed on only one occasion dealing competently with the anxious mother of a newly diagnosed child:

> 'The mother asks about school and the sister reassures her. "He'll be
> all right to go to school; he'll be treated like a normal boy and just carry
> on as normal if his diet is normal, but you'll just have to measure his
> carbohydrates – it sounds complicated but we'll teach you in stages."
> The mother asks how other parents cope. "OK", says sister, "He'll
> probably be able to do his own injections because children over 6 are
> taught to do them themselves." His mother asks about the rest of his
> life with diabetes, and sister says, "He'll always have it, but he'll
> manage, just like cleaning his teeth. He'll be able to go to school here."'

The above dialogue was by no means perfect in terms of
reassurance and support, but it did at least indicate some
acknowledgement of this particular mother's anxieties. However,
this somewhat more positive picture of the ward sister was
negated by the fact that, during this exchange, another child had
an epileptic fit in the immediate vicinity of the sister. He was
attended to by his mother and a nurse, but the event went
unremarked by the sister, who carried on with her conversation.

The transcript of the task allocation sister study contained
several examples of lack of psychosocial support:

> 'Two doctors attempt to take blood from a vein in Angela's (a 2-year-
> old Downs' Syndrome child) ankle. Sister just watches initially. She
> doesn't comfort the child, but then she puts the cotside down and
> holds the child still. The child is actually not fussing too much. The
> registrar says, "She's rather sweet, isn't she?" She is very good, in
> fact, and cries just a little when the cannula is inserted. She doesn't
> move or anything. She cries once again when the cannula is removed.
> Sister goes to get a dry swab. She comes back and holds it on the
> child's ankle while the registrar washes her hands. Sister puts the
> cotside up and asks the auxiliary to give the child some breakfast . . .
> later sister asks Nurse Grant, who is holding Angela's breakfast, to
> clean the suction apparatus at Angela's bedside.'

The transcripts of the verbal reports also did not emphasise this
type of support or attempt to identify potential problems. The
sister appeared to concentrate on the jobs to be done rather than
on the people in the ward environment. The need for support by
the nursing staff was never acknowledged and, therefore, never
addressed. However, this was not to say that other trained staff
did not acknowledge and deal with psychosocial distress. A staff
nurse was heard to explain to an older auxiliary nurse that she had

sent a young auxiliary nurse to the mortuary with a bereaved mother to see a dead child, because the young auxiliary knew the mother and child well. The older auxiliary became rather alarmed about this and suggested that it was unwise because the young auxiliary might become upset and cry. The staff nurse explained that she felt that that kind of demonstration of emotion could be helpful for both the mother and the auxiliary.

DISCUSSION AND SUMMARY

Pembrey (1978), in her study of the management styles of 50 ward sisters, came to the conclusion that the nine sisters identified as 'managers' would achieve individualised patient care on their wards, because they moved through a specific management cycle (assessing, prescribing, allocating and extracting accountability for the work), which was carried out by the sister doing a round of the patients, providing written and verbal work prescriptions, allocating the nurses and extracting accountability reports for them. Pembrey also stated that these 'manager' sisters greatly differentiated their role from those of the rest of the ward staff by managing, rather than delivering, the nursing care.

Examples of non-role differentiation given by Pembrey (1980, pp.52–53) of sisters who were defined as 'non-managers' and were, therefore, assumed not to produce individualised care for the patients, are as follows:

> 'Works alone on work that could be delegated to any, or some of the team; no role differentiation:
>   Unskilled work
>   Distributes food
>   Gives primary care to patients
>   Gives technical care to patients
>   Gives medicines to patients
>
> Interacts with patients and nurses on a social non-specific, level, no role differentiation:
>   Talks with patients
>   Talks with nurses'

An example of Pembrey's (1980, p.53) view of high role differentiation is as follows:

> 'Some aspects of formal communication are unique to the role of the ward sister and can only be received or handed on by her, other

aspects of formal communication can be delegated to trained staff; high role differentiation:
Reports to nurses
Teaches nurses
Writes nursing reports
Observes patients'

The patient allocation sister in this present study engaged in all the activities described by Pembrey's 'management cycle', but, in addition, she also engaged in a great deal of social interaction with the patients, in the course of delivering technical/basic care or for sociable reasons alone. This was one of the major means by which she demonstrated her conceptualisation of the patients as individuals rather than as a series of tasks. This was reflected in the nature of the interaction between most of the remaining nursing staff, and emphasised the importance of the ward sister as a role model.

Pembrey (1980, p.52) appeared to ignore this aspect of the ward sister in her research and stated that:

'During data collection for the main study, it was observed that the majority of Sisters did not fulfil the managerial aspects of their role and, further, that a number of them did not appear to differentiate their role from that of the trained nurse, the trainee or even the nursing auxiliary; that is, a number of sisters spent the majority of their discretionary time, not on the identification, specification and organisation of nursing, but on the delivery of nursing.'

Pembrey appeared to be suggesting that sisters should not engage in the delivery of nursing care, but should distance themselves by a hierarchical arrangement of work, in which the patient appears as an object to be 'managed'. This has serious implications for nurse education (is it really necessary in its present form?), and even more serious implications for standards of nursing care, if the ward sister is to distance herself, to a large extent, from the centrality of nursing in order to provide a 'manager' role model for the rest of the trained staff. This could result in the actual nursing care of patients becoming the province of the untrained.

The patient allocation sister in the present study both managed and delivered the nursing care. She probably fell between the two extremes of role differentiation and non-differentiation. She conceptualised her work in terms of the people involved rather than the tasks (management or otherwise) that it generated, and this, in turn, informed the nature of her interaction with the patients and the way in which she organised the work. Pembrey (1980) admitted that she did not investigate whether the patients in the wards run by the nine 'manager' sisters actually received individualised care, or even what this care looked like or how it was practised. Neither could she say whether it constituted 'good nursing care'.

There still remained the possibility that the 'manager' sisters could conceptualise the patients as a series of tasks, particularly since the types of role model these sisters were portraying were ones concerned with jobs such as ward rounds and reports and not engaging in non-specific (whatever that may mean) social interaction with the patients.

It would appear, in the present study, that it was the patient-centredness of the sister that was important, rather than her particular management style. The patient allocation sister was aware of her own significance, in terms of being inclusive with regard to the patients as described by Coser (1963).

Because the patient allocation sister was patient orientated in her day-to-day behaviour on the ward, it was likely that her power as a role model would pervade and influence the behaviour of the staff under her control in relation to their interaction with the patients and their families. The notion of this reproduction of social behaviour will be examined in the section covering the child studies.

By way of contrast, the task allocation sister demonstrated high role differentiation and performed most of the items that construct Pembrey's management cycle. She, however, conceptualised her work in terms of a series of tasks, and this was, in turn, reflected in the nature of the interaction between the nurses and the patients. There appears to be more to the production of individualised care than just good management. Maybe it was the nature of the people, rather than the procedures that they carried out, that was crucial.

The task allocation sister did not demonstrate any awareness of her own importance in creating her role; instead, her interests focused on the constraints and limitations to her work, rather than on the possibilities and challenges.

This section of the study has examined in some detail what the ward sisters actually did. Some assertions have been made regarding the possible effects of the sisters' behaviour on the activities of the rest of the staff and, thus, the experiences of the patients while in hospital.

The chapter on the experiences of four children will provide evidence to support these assertions. Although the sisters' activities were chronicled in great detail, it was not possible, within the existing research design framework, to examine the reasons for the difference in work conceptualisations demonstrated by each of them. This would clearly be a useful progression for future research in relation to a study of this kind.

4 | The hospital experiences of sick children

INTRODUCTION

It will be remembered, from the discussion of the research methods in chapter 2, that a total of 11 children from each of the two wards was observed in detail, from the point of admission up to a maximum of 4 days' hospital stay. Because of the large amount of data that this type of research method generated, it was decided to select four children (two from each ward) for the purpose of examining their admission and their subsequent hospital stay. The analysis will focus on evidence of patient-/task-centredness and psychosocial support.

Each child was paired with a similar child on the other ward. The similarities were in terms of age or diagnostic category/cultural background. These two pairs of children consisted of two Asian girls and two asthmatic boys. The experiences of the two Asian girls will be discussed first. Both of these children were of a similar age and had been in this country for only a short time. Consequently both had a language difficulty.

BALBINDER AND THE PATIENT ALLOCATION WARD

Balbinder was admitted to the patient allocation ward at 15.55 hrs on a Monday. She was 8 years old and was observed for the maximum period of 4 days.

The reason for admission was painful swelling of her finger and toe joints. She was accompanied by her uncle, who acted as an interpreter.

Admission

Balbinder was examined by the house physician, who was accompanied by a nurse. Great care was taken to screen the bed while the doctor examined the child's abdomen (the bed did not have integral screens – portable screens were wheeled to the bedside).

As the child did not speak English, questions by the doctor or nursing staff were relayed through the child's uncle. The nurse asked the doctor if the child needed to be confined to bed. The doctor thought that the child might not be too comfortable walking around, but suggested showing her where the toilet was. When the doctor left, the nurse brought two chairs for the use of the child's uncle and herself.

A state enrolled nurse came and asked if the child would like something for tea; she requested tea and cake. The student nurse elicited the child's personal details from her uncle. While this was being carried out, the child sat quietly in bed eating her tea.

The child had not been in hospital before, or away from home for that matter; she was a vegetarian, and her uncle wanted to know whether food could be brought in. The nurse said this was possible, but she assured him that the hospital was able to provide special food too.

The child apparently slept with her mother and did not go to school. She had been in this country about 7 months and could not go to school until she had had some injections. The uncle requested the hospital telephone number, which the nurse supplied, written on a piece of paper, telling him to ring up any time 'night or day'. The SEN asked if the child wanted sugar in her tea. The admitting nurse discussed with the uncle any visitors for the rest of the day (no-one else was coming), and she ensured that the child understood about that.

When the child's uncle had gone, the nurse used words and gestures to find out if the child wanted to use the lavatory. She did, so the nurse offered to carry her in case it hurt her to walk. After carrying the child to the lavatory, the nurse closed the door and waited outside to ensure privacy. The child was then carried back to bed. The nurse placed a bed-table over the bed for the cup of tea, and tried to explain that the tea was hot; she covered the child with a small blanket because she was lying outside the bedclothes. She then left the child in order to attend to another patient. This marked the end of the admission procedure. There were several significant omissions, inasmuch as the child's baseline observations, e.g. temperature, weighing and measuring, were not seen to be monitored. However, the urine, which the child passed in the lavatory, was saved for testing. This evidence could suggest a variety of ideas. The nurse was obviously not constrained by the routine aspects of the admission. She was prepared to be opportunist in the collection of the baseline data. Perhaps she felt it was more important for the child to enjoy her tea than to be bothered with these rather irritating procedures. The admission itself was carried out thoughtfully and with attention to the child's individual needs. Two nurses interacted with the child during the admission; one of these was a trained nurse. Both nurses addressed their conversation directly to the child, while the uncle interpreted.

Although not addressed for the purpose of this book, a detailed analysis of the admission experiences of all 22 child study children was carried out (Brown, 1986). The score achieved for Balbinder's admission, using the detailed analysis, was considered to be good.

SURINDER AND THE TASK ALLOCATION WARD

Surinder was 9 years old. She was admitted to the task allocation ward, also on a Monday, at 12.20 hrs, for investigations of congenital heart disease and cerebral abscess. She was observed for a total of 3 days, and was accompanied on admission by her parents and an uncle. The family had arrived in the UK just over 6 weeks earlier.

Admission

When first seen, the child was sitting with her family in the special unit attached to the ward. She had just vomited and her mother was attempting to clean the child with some tissues, which she had been given by Nurse Shaw. Nurse Mountford was also present. Both nurses left to obtain other cleaning materials. Nurse Shaw returned with a mop and bucket and lifted the child to another chair while she cleaned the floor.

It was difficult to establish the sex of this child, as she had short hair and was wearing brown trousers; however, she also had nail polish on her finger and toenails. Nurse Shaw took the mop away and returned with Nurse Mountford, who asked the child if she was feeling better. She then told the relatives that she would weigh *him*.

The child was weighed and measured by the nurses. They offered to carry her to the scales, but her father, who spoke good English, did this and interpreted the instructions to her. Nurse Shaw called her 'a good lad'!

The family were shown to Surinder's bed by the nurses, and, again, the child was carried by her father. Both nurses involved themselves in collecting the baseline technical data (temperature etc.). Questions were asked about language difficulty, previous admissions and dietary restrictions (the child did not eat beef). Nurse Shaw explained about the doctor coming to see the child later, and said that visiting was until 20.00 hrs, with the concession that they could visit later if visiting earlier was difficult. She offered to get the family some chairs and the hospital telephone number. She also explained about the name of the ward.

Nurse Shaw attempted to engage the child in conversation about speaking English because her father had explained earlier that she could understand a little if speech was slow, as all the family had been learning. However, the child was too miserable to respond. The child declined the nurses' offer of books and a drink of water. Nevertheless, the nurses returned with these items, despite the fact that the father explained that a drink of orange squash had made Surinder sick in the first place. The nurse persisted:

'A glass of water just sipped might be OK.'

Nurse Shaw adjusted the child's backrest so that she could lie down, and explained about the toilet facilities. She then left the family quietly chatting together.

The child, although not obviously distressed, appeared miserable and unwell during the admission. This was exacerbated by the vomiting episode. Despite this, the routines of the admission appeared to be adhered to, e.g. weighing, measuring, temperature taking, etc., and much was made of cleaning the floor while the mother attended to the child.

The 'nurse knows best' attitude appeared to prevail in the drink situation, although it seemed that the child just wanted to be left alone to rest. She was not asked if she wanted to go to the toilet, only told what to do if she wanted to pass urine.

It was understood from the kardex entry that this child was admitted with a history of frontal headache for 3 days and a period of unconsciousness at 08.15 hrs on the day of admission. Part of her diagnosis was ?cerebral abscess. In these circumstances, the offer of a bedpan would have been more appropriate, as would have been the omission of books to read.

However, the task allocation nurse was flexible in her approach to visiting hours, and was prepared to give information about the doctor's visit, the ward name and the hospital telephone number.

The conversation that the nurse had with the child about speaking English was unhelpful inasmuch as the nurse appeared to be merely confirming that the child could not understand. No further efforts were made to compensate for the child's language problems, either during the admission period or during the subsequent hospital stay.

The score achieved for this admission was considered to be average for a task allocation ward admission.

Discussion

The admissions of the two Asian girls tended to confirm the earlier analysis of child admissions (Brown, 1986) in that the patient allocation nurses were more patient-centred, with attention being given to the total physical and psychosocial needs of the family unit. There was an increased trained staff involvement in the admission process on the patient allocation ward. The approach to admissions on the task allocation ward was more task orientated, with no evidence of trained staff involvement.

BALBINDER'S AND SURINDER'S HOSPITAL EXPERIENCES

It will be recalled, from the discussion of the research methodology in chapter 2, that a system of time sampling was used in the observation of the children. Using this method, it was possible to construct a profile of each of the children's activities and interactions.

As observations of the children were a combination of timed 5-minute observations (divided into 10-second intervals) and diary records, it was necessary to analyse them differently.

Each 10-second observation was counted as a single observation, as was the observation of the child during the general ward
study. Using this method, the patient allocation child (Balbinder)
was observed for a total of 992 times and the task allocation child
(Surinder) for a total of 682 times. The discrepancy between these
two figures is explained by the fact that Surinder was transferred
to another ward after 3 days and that she was also absent from the
ward, undergoing tests, for two of the observation periods. Using
the activity code previously described in chapter 2, it was possible
to construct an overview of the children's activities (table 8).

Table 8   Asian girls' 10-second observations

		Patient allocation: Balbinder		Task allocation: Surinder	
		n	%	n	%
Total observations		992	100	682	100
Position of child	Bed	762	77	599	88
	Up	172	17	–	–
	Carried	6	1	–	–
	Mobile	52	5	83	12
Activity level	1. (asleep)	31	3	102	15
	2. (awake, unobservant)	–	–	52	8
	3. (awake, observant)	410	41	260	38
	4. (active)	551	56	268	39
Interacting with:	Nurses	205	21	17	2
	Visitors	107	11	362	53
	Doctors	45	5	30	4
	Patients	47	5	–	–
	Other staff	–	–	–	–
Mood	Contented	958	97	580	85
	Happy	3	0	–	–

N.B. Figures 0.5 and above have been rounded up; those below 0.5 have
been rounded down.

Because the unit of analysis was a 10-second interval, including the observation of the child during the ward study (which also took approximately 10 seconds to complete), the figures shown in table 8 are able to convey some idea of the amount of time that the nurses spent with these two small girls.

Interaction with the nurses

On the patient allocation ward, a nurse was present with Balbinder for 21% of the observations. On the task allocation ward, a nurse was present for only 2% of the observations, a difference of 19%, which is fairly substantial. It could be argued that the nurse will tend to be in the patient's company in the absence of the parents, and there was a greater parental presence in Surinder's case (362 observations with parents present). However, on a closer examination of the data, it was found that the nurses' and parents' presence with the child on the task allocation ward coincided on nine occasions of 10-second observation, while on the patient allocation ward, the parents were observed to be present for only two of the observations during which there was a nurse present. It would seem, therefore, that there was more interaction during the presence of parents on the task allocation ward and less on the patient allocation ward. Perhaps this is an indication of an increased awareness on the patient allocation ward of the child's psychosocial needs when the parents are absent.

The analytical style that was used for the ward sister study was repeated for the child study diaries – that is, interactions initiated by others with the child were categorised according to identity of interactor and purpose of interaction. It should be noted that instances of the child as initiator were not considered to be of sufficient quantity to necessitate separate analysis. In fact, the task allocation child was not observed to initiate interaction with nurses at all. It was difficult to analyse content of interaction with relatives due to the language barrier, and it was also, therefore, impossible to designate the initiator of the interaction in these circumstances – it was possible only to state that interaction was taking place. The time-sampling method did not facilitate the identity of initiators if interaction was already in progress at the beginning of the observation period. Despite these difficulties, it was possible to discern that the patient allocation child initiated interaction on three occasions with the nurses, compared with no initiated interactions with nurses by the task allocation child. One occasion of patient-initiated interaction on the patient allocation ward concerned Balbinder indicating food in her locker to a nurse, who was going around the ward collecting up edibles that parents had left for their children. This is an interesting little vignette, inasmuch as it concerns a routine that is probably endemic to many children's wards in this country, and it was obviously a routine that this particular child became aware of after a relatively short time as an in-patient (4½ hours).

Although the patient allocation child was observed for 4 days and the task allocation child observed for 3, it was possible to disregard this difference of the one day by dealing with the numbers of interactions in terms of percentages and proportions of the whole.

It will be noted from table 9 that on the patient allocation ward there was a total of 45 interactions initiated by others; of these, 32 (72%) were initiated by nurses. Nine of these interactions were for sociable reasons. In contrast, on the task allocation ward, of a total of 41 interactions initiated by others, 14 (34%) were initiated by nurses. Of these, three were for sociable reasons.

On a quantitative level, the interaction on the patient allocation ward does not appear to be greater than that on the task allocation ward. However, these figures could be misleading unless the

Table 9 Interactions initiated by others with the Asian girls

		Patient allocation: Balbinder		Task allocation: Surinder	
		n	%	n	%
Nurses	Auxiliaries	4	9	2	5
	Learners	16	36	12	29
	Trained	12	27	–	–
Others	Doctors	4	9	7	18
	Visitors	7	15	18	44
	Other children	2	4	1	2
	Visiting nursing officer	–	–	1	2
	Total	45	100	41	100

content of the interactions is examined in qualitative terms, i.e. the nine occasions of sociable interaction noted on the patient allocation ward may have involved nine occasions when nurses merely said 'Hello' to the child, and the three occasions noted on the task allocation ward may have involved nurses engaging in long episodes of good quality sociable interaction with the child. An examination of the content of the interaction has shown that the patient allocation nurses made much effort to relate to the child on a sociable basis, with emphasis on play and learning English words. By the end of the fourth day's observations, Balbinder was able to engage in competent verbal communication with those around her. In contrast, the communication of the task allocation child was not facilitated in this way, and she remained handicapped in relation to the language gap.

Interaction with the trained staff

During the analysis of the ward sister study, it was hypothesised that if the sister interacted with the children in all categories, but particularly on a sociable basis, this would be reflected in the level of interaction by the learners, who, according to Briggs (1972), provide 75% of all bedside nursing care. There appears to be some support for this, in that, on the patient allocation ward, the trained staff were responsible for 27% of the total interactions initiated by others with Balbinder (see table 9), of which 7% were for sociable reasons. On the task allocation ward, there was only one interaction recorded by a trained nurse, who was the visiting unit nursing officer and, therefore, not a member of the ward staff (this interaction has been recorded in a separate category in table 9).

Interaction and basic care

While table 9 shows that the patient allocation nurses interacted more with the patient, further examination shows that a higher proportion of interactions was related to a delivery of basic care, i.e. 59% (19) for patient allocation, compared with 50% (7) for task allocation (table 10). This would tend to support the claims made by the professional ideology that patient allocation facilitates the delivery of better basic care. It could be argued that the patient allocation child needed more basic care than did the task allocation child. However, the children's basic care needs were similar, as were their dependency levels. It could also be argued that this type of research method was recording numbers of interactions rather than evaluating quality of care. Nevertheless, it was noted by the researcher that the basic care observed was competently carried out, and it was clear that the patient allocation child actually received more basic care than the task allocation child. What is more, some of this care was given by trained staff, which was not the case on the task allocation ward. (There were six interactions by trained staff on the patient allocation ward in relation to basic care, but none on the task allocation ward; see table 10.)

Number of nurses interacting

The professional ideology postulates that one of the perceived advantages of patient allocation is that the patient interacts with fewer nurses, who will be able to develop a less superficial social relationship with him/her. Thus, nurses become more aware of that patient's individuality and uniqueness.

From the analysis of these two child studies, evidence began to emerge that would appear to contradict the above notion in terms of numbers of nurses interacting. It would seem that in a situation of task allocation, the patient received the nurses' attention only in relation to some of the tasks that needed to be performed (the task allocation child received less basic care than the patient allocation child). The nurses did not appear to engage socially with the patients on occasions other than these, whereas most of the staff on the patient allocation ward appeared to relate to most of the patients (regardless of individual allocations) on occasions other than those associated with the tasks to be performed.

In brief, the number of nurses interacting with the patients on the task allocation ward was less than those interacting on the patient allocation ward (7 nurses over a 3-day period on the task allocation ward, 13 over a 4-day period on the patient allocation ward). For the first 3 days, the patient allocation child interacted with 10 different nurses. Sociable interaction appears to be increased in the latter situation, not only in terms of quality and quantity of interactions, but also in terms of the number of personnel willing to engage in sociable interactions with any one patient. The researcher did not include data on staffing levels during the observation of the admission period. However, accurate information relating to the availability of potential staff

Table 10 Interaction by nurses in relation to basic care: Asian girls and asthmatic boys

Patient allocation

Balbinder

	n	%
Nurse interactions	32	100
Basic care interactions		
Auxiliary	3	9
Learners	10	31
Trained	6	19
Total basic care interactions	19	59

James

	n	%
Nurse interactions	52	100
Basic care interactions		
Auxiliary	1	
Learners	11	
Trained	5	
Total basic care interactions	17	33

Task allocation

Surinder

	n	%
Nurse interactions	14	100
Basic care interactions		
Auxiliary	2	14
Learners	5	36
Trained	–	–
Total basic care interactions	7	50

Laurie

	n	%
Nurse interactions	24	100
Basic care interactions		
Auxiliary	1	
Learners	1	
Trained	2	
Total basic care interactions	4	17

interactors was available for the period of the children's hospital stay.

On the patient allocation ward, Balbinder interacted with a total of 13 different nurses over the 4-day observation period. This figure was calculated by noting nurse interactions and reasons for interaction recorded during the 10-second observations, the diary recordings and the ward study. Of these staff, five were trained nurses and two auxiliaries. The remaining seven were learners. These nurse interactors and the reasons for their interactions are summarised in table 11. The staff marked with asterisks are those who were allocated to care for Balbinder. Nurse McNair was allocated to her the most often – the afternoon and evening of day one, the morning and afternoon of day two, the afternoon and evening of day three and the morning of day four. This evidence tends to support the patient allocation sister's assertion, in the interview, that she attempted to maintain some continuity in the allocation of nurses to patients. Nurse Potts was allocated for the morning of day three and the sister in charge, Sister Bottomly, took a turn in caring for this child for the afternoon and evening of day four.

It will be noted that there was considerable involvement of the trained staff in the care of this child in terms of interaction for both basic and sociable reasons. In a more hierarchical setting, it is more likely that any trained staff interaction, where it existed, would be related to technical matters.

The amount of sociable interaction was surprising in itself in view of the 'busy-ness' of the ward, and says much for the motivation and priorities of the staff, who found time to concentrate on sociability alone without the supposed incentive of a job to be done.

Earlier research (Fretwell, 1978) found evidence to suggest that nurses thought that basic care was boring, unrewarding and unconducive to learning, but in this particular instance, with this particular patient and these particular nurses, basic care dominated the care scene. This point was made earlier, using a different method of data analysis (number of 10-second observations rather than number of interactions involving nurses). The information regarding these nurse-related interactions – used to identify numbers of different interactors – was gathered from the individual child study diaries; the ward study was also inspected for nurse interactions. Finally, the staff

Table 11 Numbers of nurse interactors on both wards

Nurses	Reason for interaction				Total
	Basic	Technical	Social	Administration	
Number of patient allocation interactors (n = 13)					
Sister Simpson (night duty)		1			1
Sister Bottomly*		1	3	1	5
Sister Duncan	1				1
S/N Bilson	3		1		4
SEN Cornwall	3				3
N Northbridge			1		1
N Philips	1				1
N McNair*	5		4	1	10
N Potts*	2		1		3
N Roberts		1			1
N Taylor	3	1			4
A/N night duty	1				1
A/N Francis	2		1		3
Total	21	4	11	2	38
Number of task allocation interactors (n = 7)					
N Shaw	3		2	1	6
N Mountford		2			2
N Prouse	1				1
N Emberton			1		1
N Garner	1				1
A/N Robinson	1				1
A/N Lester	1				1
Total	7	2	3	1	13

* allocated nurses

ward study sheets were scanned for personnel who had not already been mentioned; this was done carefully since it was possible for a member of staff to appear on both child and staff ward study sheets, with some duplication of data. This demonstrated the data compatibility when the analytical method was triangulated. It was important to establish whether or not this was so with other child studies. If it was, some credibility might be lent to the idea that 'basic care' (which is of particular importance to the patient) becomes less boring and routine if the nurse is able to conceptualise her work in terms of individual patients, rather than in terms of tasks to be completed.

On the task allocation ward, Surinder interacted with a total of seven nurses over the 3-day observation period. None of these was a trained nurse. Although Sister Albut was observed standing by Surinder's bed with the medical ward round, this was not included, as she was not interacting with Surinder. Two of the interactors were auxiliary nurses and the remaining five were learners. The distribution of interactions in relation to nurse and content is depicted in table 11.

No-one was specially responsible for Surinder's care, and she did not form part of a block allocation. The staff listed in table 11 were allocated tasks on the work list, e.g. Nurse Shaw: bedmaking and responsibility for two children on intravenous drip feeds. Auxiliary Nurse Lester was listed to look after a mentally retarded child who required frequent basic care, for the serving of suppers and for the locker round.

The figures are striking in terms of lowness in comparison with the patient allocation ward. It was felt that the low figures could not be accounted for by the reduced observation time of 3 days (there were also two observation schedules omitted from the third day of Surinder's study because the child went for X-ray). Even if these figures were increased by 25%, they still would not reach the level of the patient allocation ward in terms of number of nurses or number of interactions.

It could be argued that the reduced observation time could considerably affect the number of potential and actual interactors on the task allocation ward. However, the number of potential nurse interactors was exactly the same for the two wards, i.e. 22 nurses were available for interaction on the patient allocation ward, over 4 days, and 22 on the task allocation ward over 3 days. The number of actual interactors with the patient allocation child was counted for the first 3 days of her stay, to bring her in line with Surinder. For this reduced time, Balbinder was interacting with 10 different nurses while Surinder interacted with seven. Again, it could be argued that the loss of two schedules from the observations on Surinder would affect this, but it is unlikely that two more observations would have produced three more nurse interactors.

JAMES AND THE PATIENT ALLOCATION WARD

Two further children were selected for analysis and discussion of their admission and subsequent hospital experience. The choice was made on the grounds that both were 9 years old, had experienced previous hospital admission and belonged to the same diagnostic category. Laurie, on the task allocation ward, was admitted as a poorly controlled asthmatic for assessment. James, on the patient allocation ward, was admitted with acute asthma, and could be considered to be rather more ill on admission than Laurie.

Admission

James had a long history of asthma. His kardex entry relating to his past medical history stated:

'Was in fairly good health until 3 years of age, although he was noticed to be quite chesty on and off. Started wheezing at 3 years of age. Has had three previous admissions with asthma. Also has eczema on face, backs of legs and groins. He is prescribed steroid cream for this, which Mum applies when necessary. Mum can't remember name of cream.'

There was also a comprehensive account of his present medical history, his condition on admission and his social history, which included:

'James is a quiet, shy boy who needs a lot of encouragement to talk. Does not want to mix with other children at the moment. Mother divorced – lives with boyfriend. Youngest child; brother 17 years, sister 12 years. Likes drinking chocolate, Ribena, tea and coke. Eats most things, likes spaghetti.'

This report was written on the normal proforma used by the whole hospital. Previously, this ward had used the normal kardex with additional headings printed on it, in order to include the child's personal preferences and evidence of uniqueness. However, since the ward had had to pay for these additions, they had been discontinued when the ward could no longer afford the financial outlay. This reversal back to the orthodox kardex did not appear to have prevented this particular nurse from acknowledging James's individuality.

During the admission procedure it was interesting to observe how James used his illness to manipulate his mother into providing indulgent luxuries. This was precipitated by his mother promising him a new car if he was a good boy; later he asked:

> '... if the shops are open today. "What for?", says his mum. "The car", he says ... Nurse Marshall asks him about his present illness. He tells her it started last night and then he hides his face in his mother's chest. His mother says she will get him a car. "Tonight?", he says. "Yes, I will send it in". "Any sweets?", he asks. "Only Polos in my bag." ... His mother talks to him and he goes on about getting a car. He wants her to go and buy one now and come back with it. She agrees and goes ... He tells the nurse about his mother going to get a car. His mother later returned with a whole new cabinet of dinky toys with 45 different models in it!'

The routine/technical aspects of the admission were competently carried out, i.e. weighing, measuring, temperature assessment and urinalysis. Additionally, the nurse took a great interest in both the physical and psychosocial needs of the family unit. She asked about James's Christmas presents, explained about the bath for big boys and about not having to stay in the side ward if he wanted to go and watch TV with the other children when he felt better. She took an interest in his family background and got him his favourite drink, having established his personal preferences in terms of diet, leisure activities, etc.

The nurse's attention to comfort detail was phenomenal, e.g. she closed the curtains so that the TV picture was clearer. She also used strategies to reduce distancing between herself and the family unit, such as sitting on the floor while they sat in chairs, talked about her birthday and James's both being in September, and, when the mother passed a comment about James's feet smelling, the nurse said it was probably hers!

There was trained staff involvement, inasmuch as Sister Bottomly not only acknowledged the family but made particular reference to their family circumstances:

> 'Sister Bottomly chats to the mother as she goes into the side ward. She tells James that she has seen his big brother, who is a diabetic and has been circumcised and has also lost his job. Sister Morgan joins in the discussion ... James's mother tells Sister Bottomly that she is working at Asda. Sister says, "Oh you can get us things cheap." She then asks about James's brother's daily insulin.'

The admitting nurse also used strategies to establish some

continuity between home and hospital. These strategies also had a familiarising quality:

> 'The nurse talks about school. "You can go to school here", she says – he's not keen but he likes painting.'

Initially, the child looked anxious and ill at ease. However, this seemed to resolve itself to the point that he was appreciating jokes made by the nurse:

> 'The nurse says, "Would you like a drink?" "Drinking chocolate", he says. The nurse asks about other drinks he likes and says jokingly, "Beer?"'

The nurse showed James the nearest toilet, the TV set in the main ward, the playroom where he could eat if he wanted to and the selection of toys, from which he made a choice. She gave him the opportunity of various options – a crucial element of self-determination, which is more powerful when founded on an accurate knowledge base.

As was evidenced by the information in the kardex, this child's social background was slightly unconventional, i.e. mother divorced, living with boyfriend. The nurse, however, did not refer to this, although she would have been aware of it. This appeared to be a sensitive approach, which preserved certain dimensions of family privacy.

On the whole, this admission could not be faulted in the way in which the nurse maintained the individual integrity of the patient. In relation to the admission rating scale, this admission was considered to be excellent.

LAURIE AND THE TASK ALLOCATION WARD

Laurie also had a long history of asthma; his admission kardex reported that he was:

> 'Admitted as a day case – to stay to try and control asthma. Past medical history – known asthmatic with multiple allergies to dust and pollen. Drugs commenced – salbutamol inhalations and prednisolone 15 mg. On admission, a very obese boy but quite cheerful – not breathless.'

Admission

The ward was quite busy when Laurie was admitted. Three children were being discharged and five new patients were being admitted. This entailed a great deal of cleaning, changing and moving beds and cots. This activity tended to preoccupy the staff. Laurie and his mother were left standing in the ward doorway for approximately 10 minutes, during which time the beds were being reorganised. However, staff nurse did call out:

'Be with you in a second, haven't forgotten you.'

No-one offered them a seat. They were eventually allocated a bed. The initial interaction between the patient and the hospital was related to the medical students, who spent some time with Laurie and his mother in order to complete the medical admission details. This appeared to be done sensitively with reference to the child's social identity, e.g. school life and the Boys' Brigade.

After the completion of the medical admission, the child and his mother went to the playroom. They had arrived on the ward at 14.25 hrs and it was then 15.40 hrs. On their return, his mother asked the researcher if Laurie could have a drink because he had missed the drinks trolley. The researcher passed this request on to the nurse who was going to admit Laurie – Nurse Chanelle. His mother winked at the researcher with satisfaction at this negotiation taking place. Nurse Chanelle asked about both food and drink. She provided a milk shake and then went off to have her own tea before completing the admission procedure. However, on her return, there were three doctors at Laurie's bedside, so, she did not manage to get to him until 16.30 hrs in order to complete the official admission procedure. Perhaps this procedure constitutes an important *rite de passage* for the task allocation ward staff, since this child did not appear to be treated as one of the legitimate ward population until his admission procedure had been completed.

As in the previously described admission of Surinder, much emphasis appeared to be given to the admission routines – weighing, measuring, temperature taking. The weighing and measuring aspects were not checked by a second nurse.

Although the nurse established that the child had been in hospital before, she seemed to use this information for justifying not familiarising the child with the current environment.

'You know your way around the ward – don't you?'

She made no attempt to interact with the child socially and made no offer of diversional therapy in the form of toys, books or where to find them. She offered no information to the mother except for the following mother-initiated exchange:

> 'His mother asks about pyjamas because they haven't brought any in; the nurse says she will get some and his mother says she will bring his own tomorrow. The nurse says it's OK for older children to wear their own clothes because they don't lose them like the little ones.'

The nurse seemed to be legitimating the mother's offer to bring in Laurie's own pyjamas by indicating that older children are able to be responsible for their own belongings. At no time did the nurse demonstrate her awareness of this child's uniqueness. While she was weighing and measuring Laurie, another child was sitting in the doorway weeping miserably, but the nurse did not acknowledge this misery.

On the whole, this admission seemed to be technical and task orientated and was considered poor.

Discussion

When comparing Laurie's and James's admission experiences, it would appear that James's was much more individualised and patient-centred. It may be argued that an individualised approach to patients may considerably threaten the patient's personal autonomy. Webb (1981) recognised this when she used Bernstein's (1975) code theory to analyse the change from a task-orientated to a patient-orientated mode of organisation of nursing care. In this analysis, she stated that:

> 'Areas which formerly did not enter into the treatment of the body now become available for treatment of the person. It is much more difficult for him to keep hidden those areas of life which are private and which he wants to keep to himself.' (p.373)

Webb appeared to refer only to psychosocial autonomy, but, in fact, there is the possibility that the total autonomy of the patient (psychosocial and physical) could be threatened and undermined in an individualistic approach.

Both of these admission experiences support the evidence relating to the Asian girls. On the task allocation ward the admissions were mechanistic and task orientated, while those on the patient allocation ward were organic and patient-centred. On the patient allocation ward the transition from child to patient appeared to be less pronounced in terms of the nurses' perspectives and the amount of adaptation required of the children to a different role. It seemed that it was the ward rather than the children that adapted most on the patient allocation ward. On the task allocation ward this appeared to be reversed.

JAMES'S AND LAURIE'S HOSPITAL EXPERIENCES

Both of these children were observed for 4 days. Laurie (task allocation ward), however, was absent from the ward for two 5-minute observations because he went to school on the second and fourth days.

A synopsis of the observations lasting 10 seconds (including the ward study observations) over each 4-day period is given in table 12. The patient allocation child, James, was observed 992 times, while the task allocation child, Laurie, was observed 930 times. It will be remembered that the children were observed in relation to their position, activity level, mood and with whom they were interacting.

Interaction with the nurses

As will be noted from table 13, there were more observations in which nurses were interacting with the child on the patient allocation ward; this supports the data from the observations of the Asian girls.

The fact that the disparity was not so great in the case of Laurie and James could be accounted for by the fact that Laurie (task allocation) was extremely sociable and would seek nurses out to talk to them; further evidence of this can be found in Laurie's 'position' category (see table 12) and 'other' social actors. He was up, sitting in a chair or actually walking about, for more than 50% of the observations and he was with other children for 35% of the observations. He had a cheerful disposition and was fairly gregarious. On 13 occasions he was noted as being happy rather than being merely contented.

James, on the other hand, was a much quieter child, less

Table 12 Asthmatic boys: 10-second observations

		Patient allocation: James		Task allocation: Laurie	
		n	%	n	%
Total observations		992	100	930	100
Position of child	Bed	697	70	397	43
	Up	149	15	245	26
	Up and about	146	15	288	31
Activity level	1. (asleep)	62	6	–	–
	2. (awake, unobservant)	–	–	–	–
	3. (awake, observant)	326	33	266	29
	4. (active)	604	61	664	71
Interacting with:	Nurses	161	16	98	11
	Visitors	345	35	259	28
	Doctors	59	6	4	0
	Patients	145	15	322	35
	Other staff	1	0	3	0
Mood	Contented	897	90	917	99
	Happy	1	0	13	1
	Distressed	32	3	–	–

gregarious, and was observed to be up in a chair or walking about for 30% of the observations. He was noted with other children for 15% of the observations. James was rather more ill on admission than was Laurie, but, even so, his recovery was rapid and there were opportunities for him to fraternise. He spent more of his time lying on his bed than did Laurie, and it was, therefore, necessary for the nurses to go to him, since he did not actively seek them out. The number of nurse interactions noted is, therefore, interesting, particularly in view of the comment made by Sister Bottomly:

'It will be interesting to observe a child in the side ward, because the nurses don't go in so often.'

Table 13   10-second observations of Asian girls and asthmatic boys relating to nurse interactions

	Patient allocation ward		Task allocation ward	
	Balbinder		*Surinder*	
	n	%	*n*	%
Total observations	992	100	682	100
with nurse	205	21	17	2
	James		*Laurie*	
	n	%	*n*	%
Total observations	992	100	930	100
with nurse	161	16	98	11

James, in fact, was only in the side ward until approximately 20.00 hrs on the day of admission. The amount of nurse-initiated interaction when parents were present was reversed in the cases of these two asthmatic boys (table 14, comparison with Asian girls). This could be explained by the fact that Laurie was very mobile and was able to make himself available for interaction with the nurses when left to his own devices.

Table 14   Nurse interactions when parents were present: Asian girls and asthmatic boys

	Patient allocation		Task allocation	
	n	%	n	%
	Balbinder		*Surinder*	
Nurse interactions	205	100	17	100
Parents present	2	1	9	53
	James		*Laurie*	
Nurse interactions	161	100	98	100
Parents present	22	14	9	9

Overt somatic or psychosocial distress was not a feature of the observed experiences of the two Asian girls or of Laurie on the task allocation ward. James, however, was an exception to this, and was observed to be distressed for 32 of the 10-second observations. There are clearly disadvantages to this method of recording distress, since it conveys little information about the frequency or the length of distress episodes. It would have been possible to have accounted for the whole of this distress over a 5-minute observation period, thus indicating no further distress during the rest of the hospital stay. However, on a closer examination of the data, it was clear that the distress was distributed over time, with two episodes noted on the second day and two on the third day, when a major episode involving his mother occurred. It was also possible to locate distress experiences in the diary record.

Most of the distress tended to be the consequence of feeling miserable due to a troublesome cough that James had. One episode of misery was noted when the night sister was telling James off. She told him not to worry so much and not to cry; he was coughing and retching. He recounted to the sister the narrative about his mother's car being stolen. The sister responded by saying she supposed he was worried about that. He asked when visitors could start to come and was told 'about 9 a.m.'. This may not sound a very sympathetic handling of this sick and miserable child. The night sister was very hale and hearty and went about her work in a very noisy fashion. However, she was not unaware of James's worries and was prepared to acknowledge them. Her attitude appeared to work and James seemed more settled after she left.

The main episode of misery recorded occurred on the third day, when James's mother and aunt were present. At one point, Nurse Marshall asked what was the matter. His mother said he was feeling a bit touchy. James's tears were very intermittent. His mother threatened to go home because he was so miserable. This created more tears. His mother did little to distract or comfort him, preferring to gossip with her sister. A later conversation with his mother established that she thought James was miserable because he was put in the toddler section of the ward at approximately 20.00 hrs on the day of admission, although subsequently he made friends with one of the Asian toddlers during the day after admission. Then he was moved into a section of the ward for older children, where he complained about being next to a girl.

However, after he had made friends with her, she was moved by the nurses into a 'girls only' section and James felt bereft of friends (the children left in this section were a 12-year-old boy whose behaviour was sometimes anti-social because of brain damage, and a 6-year-old boy whom James possibly considered too young; the remaining bed was empty).

Moving James away from the babies and then segregating the sexes did not seem to have been in the spirit of good psychosocial support in James's case. Added to this was the fact that an intravenous infusion had been commenced on James, after the observations had been concluded at 22.00 hrs on the admission day.

The data were also analysed in terms of who initiated interactions with the boys and for what purpose. A summary of this is given in table 15. It will be noted that there was a total of 52 (59%) interactions initiated by nurses on the patient allocation ward and 24 (50%) on the task allocation ward, of which 13 (15%) on the patient allocation ward and five (10%) on the task allocation ward were for sociable reasons.

On the patient allocation ward, the bulk of the sociable interaction took place during the admission period. Nevertheless, it was of a fairly high quality. The task allocation sociable interaction was less in quantity, but of good quality when it did

Table 15 Interactions initiated with asthmatic boys by others

		Patient allocation James		Task allocation Laurie	
		n	%	n	%
Nurses	Auxiliaries	2	2	2	4
	Learners	33	38	15	31
	Trained	17	19	7	15
Others	Doctors	10	11	1	2
	Visitors	20	23	13	27
	Other children	6	7	10	21
	Total	88	100	48	100

occur. It is perhaps worth mentioning that Nurse McNair had been observed initially at work in the patient allocation ward caring for Balbinder. This nurse's observed interactional style was of a very high standard and she could be described as a deviant in the task allocation ward setting.

The use of percentages may be misleading in view of the fact that there were 52 nurse-initiated interactions on the patient allocation ward and 24 on the task allocation ward. This is less than half as many, which is a considerable difference. This is also reflected in the sociable category (13 for patient allocation and five for task allocation). It would appear that the patient allocation ward nurses interacted more with the children than did their task allocation counterparts, and the sociable type of interaction was also increased.

Interaction with the trained staff

When looking at who the interactors were in terms of trained and untrained staff, it was interesting to note that out of eight potential patient allocation trained staff interactors, seven were actual interactors. (However, two of these were the subject of child-initiated interactions.) On the task allocation ward, there were, again, eight potential trained staff interactors, of whom five were actual interactors, but none of these was solely child-initiated interactions. On the patient allocation ward the senior sister appeared in both analyses (Asian girl, asthmatic boy) as one of the actual interactors. On the task allocation ward the senior sister was not seen to interact with either the Asian girl or the asthmatic boy. This tends to support the view that the nurse in charge was used as a role model by the rest of the staff in terms of their interactional style with the children.

Pembrey (1978) found that the ward sisters who practised individualised care based their practice on previous ward sisters with whom they had worked in a junior capacity. It would, therefore, seem feasible that if the ward sister perceived patients as individuals rather than work objects, the rest of the staff would do likewise and would demonstrate this by increased social interaction generally and by sociable interaction specifically.

The behaviour of the ward sisters during the observation of the two boys was consistent with their earlier observed behaviour. The patient allocation sister continued to allocate herself to care for patients, e.g. on the second day she looked after Michael Russell and Jeremy Brown. On two occasions on day two she was noted carrying Jeremy around with her. The task allocation sister did not include herself on the work list. If this was compiled by another member of staff, the sister was usually allocated a job such as bedmaking or medicines, the latter being the case for day four of the observations.

Interaction and basic care

Table 10 above illustrates the interactions initiated by staff in relation to basic care. These are contrasted with the Asian girls.

This evidence tends to confirm the conclusions drawn from the analysis of the Asian girls' data, that not only was there more interaction by nurses on the patient allocation ward, but that there was more interaction for basic care reasons. This included basic care being delivered by trained staff. This should imply a good standard of care. However, Laurie fared a little better than Surinder in this respect on the task allocation ward, since there were two interactions recorded in relation to trained staff basic care.

Number of nurses interacting

It has already been mentioned that one of the assertions made by the professional ideology was that, if a patient allocation system of work organisation is used, the patient will interact with fewer nurses more frequently. In this instance, the difference between actual nurse interactors on each of the wards was minimal – patient allocation = 12 (including seven trained staff), task allocation = 14 (including five trained staff). In the analysis of the Asian girls' data, there were 13 actual interactors on the patient allocation ward (including five trained staff) and on the task allocation ward seven (no trained staff). This would tend to cast doubts on the commonly accepted view that patient allocation decreases the numbers of nurses with whom the patient interacts. It would also tend to neutralise one of the perceived weaknesses of patient allocation, that if nurses were allocated to a specific group of patients, they would tend to ignore the rest of the ward population.

Nursery nurse activity

The task allocation ward had a nursery nurse as part of its permanent staff complement (this was not so on the patient allocation ward). This nurse was not known to feature in the allocation of work on the work list. The reason for this was not determined but raises questions as to whether this was due to specificity of role or lack of it. On examining her activities in the ward study and child study data (table 16), it would appear that she spent her time mainly in sociable activities (playing with the children), with some basic nursing work.

It would have been useful to have observed how a nursery nurse would have functioned on the patient allocation ward, in relation to the different work perceptions of the patient allocation sister. The fact that the nursery nurse was not listed to do a particular job on the task allocation ward could offer some insight into what the sister saw as constituting work, i.e. that what the nursery nurse did (play with children) could not be defined as a job. This would appear to lend some support to the notion that the task allocation children were seen in terms of the things that were done to them, rather than in terms of social beings with whom others socialised. This view would, therefore, justify not including the nursery nurse on the work list.

Metcalfe's (1982) study of patient allocation on a maternity ward found that the nursery nurse's role was radically changed by the introduction of this method of work organisation:

'Problems can arise when some members of staff can, or only expect to, perform certain duties. In this study the person most affected by this problem was the nursery nurse, but similar problems could occur with other staff in different areas. Because the nursery nurse felt that she was employed to look after babies − all of them, not just some of

Table 16 Nursery nurse interactions

Total observations	14	Basic	2	Sociable (children)	8
		Miscellaneous	2		
				Sociable (staff)	1
				Sociable (both)	1

them – she took exception to being "expected" to help with the general care of the mothers.' (p.378)

It is likely that, had there been a nursery nurse employed on the patient allocation ward, she would have been included in the allocation of patients to nurses, as indeed the auxiliary nurses were, but that the children thus allocated would require little or no technical care.

SUMMARY AND DISCUSSION

The hospital experiences of the two asthmatic boys tend to confirm the findings discussed earlier. On the whole, James's experiences of hospital appear to be satisfactory, with the changing of the bed arrangements being the only apparent situation where the nurses did not seem to be aware of his preferences. However, they might be forgiven for believing that a 9-year-old boy would not be developing relationships and loyalties with toddlers and girls! (A critical analysis of stereotyping does not feature in many nurse education curricula!)

The instances of distress seemed to be adequately dealt with, despite the fact that distress could sometimes be redefined as manipulative behaviour.

James's admission experience was excellent. The quality and quantity of interaction by both trained and untrained staff were satisfactory. The technical procedures were carried out competently.

Laurie's admission experience was poor compared with James's. However, Laurie's subsequent experience on the task allocation ward was reasonable. This could partly be accounted for by the fact that he was of a cheerful disposition and gregarious; he was also able to negotiate on his own behalf. Despite this, the quantity and quality of the interaction by the nursing staff was not of the standard offered on the patient allocation ward, and there was less evidence of trained staff interaction. It is perhaps, therefore, not unsurprising that Laurie expressed a certain amount of relief when he was informed that he could go home. He was observed telling this fact to various people, including nurses, no less than 15 times over a very short period, during which he also visited the lavatory three times and had his leg pulled three times about his pleasure.

Both of these children's experiences tended to confirm the child-centredness of the patient allocation ward and the task-centredness of the task allocation ward. This appeared to result in a better experience of hospital for the patient allocation children.

The nature of the interaction between the staff and the children on the two wards was very different in both qualitative and quantitative terms. The number of interactions was greater on the patient allocation ward than on the task allocation ward. The quality was also good, particularly in terms of social interaction. On the task allocation ward there was less sociable interaction and, where it existed, it was of poor quality. There was more interaction by trained staff on the patient allocation ward than on the task allocation ward.

Interaction by nurses when parents were absent was increased in relation to the patient allocation Asian girl. On the task allocation ward there was more interaction when the parents were present (but it should be remembered that there was less interaction overall on the task allocation ward). However, this situation was reversed in relation to the asthmatic boys and can probably be explained by Laurie's gregariousness and mobility.

There was more child-initiated interaction with the nurses on the patient allocation ward than on the task allocation ward. The Asian girl on the task allocation ward was not observed to initiate interaction with the nurses at all.

There were more interactions for reasons of basic care on the patient allocation ward than on the task allocation ward. The patient allocation trained staff also interacted for this reason, while the task allocation staff tended not to. In the case of the Asian girls, a greater number of different nurses interacted on the patient allocation ward than did on the task allocation ward (figure 15), but, in relation to the asthmatic boys, the numbers were similar.

To link up with the ward sister study, the activities of the two sisters are worth singling out in relation to the child studies. The patient allocation sister was observed on several occasions interacting with the children; the quality of her sociable interaction was good. She often allocated herself patients on the allocation list and was frequently seen engaging in physical contact with the children, e.g. carrying, nursing on knee, etc. This inclusive type of interpretation of the patient allocation sister's role runs counter to

Patient allocation	Task allocation
1. Admissions good	1. Admissions average/poor
2. More interaction by nurses	2. Less interaction by nurses
3. Interaction with trained staff	3. Minimal interaction by trained staff
4. Good quality sociable interaction	4. Poor quality sociable interaction
5. More interactions initiated by children	5. Fewer interactions initiated by children
6. More individual nurses interacting with Asian girl	6. Similar numbers of individual nurses interacting on both wards with the asthmatic boys
7. More interaction for basic care	7. Less interaction for basic care
8. Interaction by trained staff for basic care	8. No interaction by trained staff for basic care

Figure 15 Experiences of Asian girls and asthmatic boys

the assertion made by Pembrey (1978, p.234) that:

'Role differentiation is a further guide to ward behaviour associated with the organisation of nursing on an individualised patient basis. Organisation of the nursing in relation to individual patients was not observed to occur when the ward sister behaved like the ward nurses and occupied a virtually non-differentiated role in the nursing team.'

This premise ignores the important distinction that *ward nurses may behave like the ward sister role model*. The role model, in turn, may be demonstrating an individualised approach to patient care. However, the patient allocation ward sister did fit Pembrey's (1978, p.235) criteria that the ward sisters who managed the nursing on an individualised patient basis:

'were among the most highly qualified academically and professionally.'

Pembrey (1978, p. 236) also noted:

> 'that the ability of the ward sister to achieve a form of nursing organisation which was flexible enough to cope with an unstable ward environment was one of the characteristics of the sisters, who managed the nursing in relation to individual patients and individual nurses.'

Of the two wards in this current study, the environment on the patient allocation ward was much more unstable than that on the task allocation ward, particularly in terms of 'busy-ness' factors relating to patient turnover, number of beds and consultants, out-patient attendances (on the ward) and child mortality rates. An example of the patient allocation sister's flexibility in relation to managing the nursing was her insistence that the nurses themselves determined the time of their coffee breaks in response to the work needs in operation at the time. The task allocation sister, on the other hand, carefully prescribed, in writing on the work list, the time at which each nurse should take her break, regardless of the activity in which she was engaged. The task allocation sister appeared to have a highly differentiated role according to Pembrey's (1978) definition vis-à-vis not behaving like the ward nurses in terms of the *jobs* that she performed. The task allocation sister never allocated herself a 'batch' of patients. Sometimes she was allocated a job if others planned the work list, e.g. bedmaking or drug rounds. She rarely interacted with the children for any reason, and for sociable reasons, hardly ever. She was never seen to engage in physical contact with a child patient, e.g. carrying, nursing. The only instance of physical contact that was noted was when visitors brought a younger sibling to the ward to visit and she took the child to show him to the Special Unit sister.

In conclusion, it would appear from an examination of both the admissions and the four child studies that the care of the patient allocation children was much more patient-centred and individualised than that of the task allocation children. As a final illustration of this, the following incidents were recorded in relation to the management of the Asian girls' nutritional needs (both children had cultural dietary restrictions):

> 'Balbinder is sitting at the table eating her lunch of fish and chips. Nigel has minced beef. He requests fish when he sees Balbinder's lunch. Nurse Potts explains to him that fish in the week is especially

for the children who don't eat meat, and that Balbinder is Muslim. Nigel says, "I don't eat meat." Balbinder is still eating. She is concentrating on the chips. She hasn't touched the fish yet. It looks like a sausage covered in batter; it's likely that she doesn't know what it is unless it's opened up for her. S/N Bilson comes and cuts the fish and says, "Perhaps she doesn't realise." The child understands now about the food and eats the fish.'

'Surinder has just been given roast beef and two vegetables for lunch. She looks at it and she and her father have a discussion. He returns the meal untouched to the lunch trolley ... Later Auxiliary Nurse Brown brings a boiled egg and bread and butter and says, "There you are, darling." '

5 | Epilogue

SUMMARY

This study was designed to determine the nature of task and patient allocation in terms of the activities of the nursing staff, particularly in relation to the quality of their interaction with the patients. The study was particularly concerned with the degree of patient-centredness present with each type of work organisation and the standard of care which thus ensued, and with whether this was, in fact, related to how work was organised.

Following a review of the literature, it became clear that there was no firm evidence to support the professional ideology that had made the assumption that patient allocation resulted in more individualised patient care. It was also difficult to ascertain what actually constituted individualised care and whether or not this resulted in improved 'quality of care'. Metcalfe (1982, p.372) stated that:

> 'When trying to assess if patient centred methods of delivering nursing care result in better quality of care being delivered, it is important to remember that if improved "quality" of care is defined in terms of the "patient centredness" of the care, then it is likely that care which is adapted to the individual needs of the patient will, by definition, be improved.'

There is a basic assumption being made in this statement that patient-centred care probably produces improved care.

However, Metcalfe (1982) does go on to suggest that her study, which examined patient and staff satisfaction in a maternity ward that had changed from task allocation to patient allocation, was not the most suitable means of assessing quality of care. She also believed that:

'It might be more useful to develop a method of assessing the quality of nursing care given on wards which have been graded as to their "degree of patient-centredness".' (pp.371–372)

This present study has attempted to define not only how patient-centred care manifested itself in terms of the nature of the interaction between the nursing staff and the patients, but also whether the quality of care was improved, in terms of how the patients experienced hospitalisation, if this style of caring philosophy was adopted.

The data for the study were obtained from two medical wards in a children's hospital. One ward was said to practise a task allocation method of work organisation and the other a patient allocation method.

The following methods were used for the collection of the data: semi-structured interviews and non-participant observation of the children and staff. The sisters, who were in overall charge of each of the two wards, were interviewed in order to obtain some idea as to whether they conceptualised their work in terms of tasks or patients. In addition, each of the ward sisters was observed for a period of 3 days, and a detailed diary account was recorded of all their activities. This was done in order to confirm how they put their work concepts into practice.

Observations of 11 specific children on each ward were carried out using a time-sampling technique. Each child was observed, on average, for a total of 80 minutes spread over a 4-hour period. This was done daily for not more than 4 days or until discharge, whichever was the shorter period. The 4-hour observation periods were arranged in order to cover the waking day over the days of the week.

In addition, a detailed diary account of each child's hospital experience was recorded. The data relating to the child's admission experience were also collected using the diary method. It was, therefore, possible to construct an accurate picture of how each child experienced the hospital, from the time of admission until discharge or until 4 days had elapsed.

THE MAJOR FINDINGS

The findings focus around the following major areas of study:

1. the work concepts of the sisters;
2. the sisters' work concepts in practice;
3. the 'quality of care' experienced by individual children.

The sisters' work concepts

From the interview with the patient allocation sister, it became clear that she conceptualised her work in terms of the patients she was caring for. She was also aware of, and concerned about, the nurses in the ward, and acknowledged her role in relation to learner supervision and teaching in order to ensure good care. She prioritised her work in terms of interaction with the patients, rather than in terms of jobs to be done. She also emphasised the teaching of the learners in order to maintain high standards of care and for the creation of a good working atmosphere. She also showed awareness of the importance of her own influence in relation to how the ward was managed (role creation). She was able to engage in constructive criticism of her own performance.

Her view of the ward in an ideal state was when the children were engaged in quiet play with no extra personnel working in the ward (as was often the case on Sunday mornings). She demonstrated an innovative approach to her work, inasmuch as she had previously experienced working in a traditional task allocation situation and had felt she wanted to do things differently. Her general and professional educational background was similar to that of Pembrey's (1978) 'manager sisters'.

By way of contrast to the patient-centredness of the patient allocation sister, the task allocation sister demonstrated a more task-orientated conceptualisation of her work role, which she saw in terms of organising the ward or seeing that the nurses were supervised and got varied experience. She did, however, go on to say that her job was also about communicating with parents, other staff and the patients. When discussing work priorities, she found it difficult to state what was most important, maintaining that everything was. She appeared to be trying to isolate a particular job rather than a specific orientation, e.g. a high level of patient satisfaction. In order to clarify this, she was asked what she would leave out – she then mentioned several tasks that, ironically, would make her available to the patients, e.g. bedmaking, serving meals, drug rounds. The patients did not, in fact, feature a great deal in her deliberations. When asked to describe the ward looking at its best, she jokingly said, 'When it's empty'. She did not see herself as a constraint or an asset in relation to how the ward was managed. In fact, she saw constraints in terms of externals over which she had no control, such as the impositions made by the nursing hierarchy, and the unpunctuality of the doctors. She was also much influenced by traditional work organisation methods. Her stated reason for running the ward as she did was because it had always been done that way.

The sisters' work concepts in practice

The patient allocation sister spent more time interacting with the children and their families, both in relation to specific basic and technical nursing care and in terms of sociable interaction, than did the task allocation sister. Not only was this true in quantitative terms, but also in terms of the quality of the interaction. Evidence has shown that the patient allocation ward was much busier than the task allocation ward, and it could be argued that the patient allocation sister needed to interact more because of this factor. However, on a closer examination of the content of the interaction, the patient allocation sister demonstrated more awareness of the child population on her ward. For example, she would socialise with the children even when engaged in technical work such as medicine rounds. The task allocation sister invariably never did this. The patient allocation sister did not require nursing functions to legitimise her sociable interaction, as she often interacted on a sociable basis for its own sake. Conversely, it could be argued that, because the task allocation ward was less busy, the task allocation sister had more time and, therefore, more opportunity to interact with the children and their families, but this was not so. If the task allocation sister had no reason to be in the patient area, e.g. for doctors' or drug rounds, she withdrew to her office. It appeared that any sociable interaction initiated by her needed to be legitimated by some task she was performing for the patient.

The two sisters were very different in their management of the physical environment, particularly in relation to their use of space. The patient allocation sister used the facilities on the ward for the benefit of the children and their families, and was instrumental in the provision of psychosocial support as well as physical comfort and convenience. The task allocation sister had available similar accommodation, which was under-utilised.

The patient allocation sister demonstrated more awareness of the psychosocial needs of everyone (patients, relatives and staff) than did the task allocation sister. Verbal reports on the patient allocation ward tended to focus on the children's total needs as individuals, while the reports on the task allocation ward tended to discuss the children almost exclusively in terms of the technical aspects of their care, in relation to the medical treatment that they were currently receiving.

One of the striking features of the patient allocation sister was the way in which she integrated her work with that of the ward team. While she clearly acted as a co-ordinator, liaison and leader in relation to the ward staff, she did not set herself totally apart. She was frequently observed interacting with the children and engaging in low status activities such as bedmaking. She was also allocated children to care for, although perhaps not as many as the rest of the staff, and she did not highly differentiate her role from that of the ward nurses in terms of her interaction with the children and of the work that she actually did. This dimension is likely to be crucial to the level of her power as a role model, particularly in areas of an interactionist nature.

Conversely, the task allocation sister spent her time rather differently from the ward nurses because she engaged in many activities unrelated to direct patient care. Her activities with the patients were usually concerned with the high status tasks such as medicine rounds. She was sometimes observed making beds and serving meals, but these activities did not often involve direct contact with the patients. She was never observed in direct physical contact with a child patient.

These two views of the ward sister run contrary to Pembrey's (1978, p.233) notion that sisters who manage the ward on an individualised patient basis:

'highly differentiated their role from that of the ward nurses ... minimal role differentiation on the part of the sister was associated with non-management of nursing.'

Individual child studies – degrees of quality of care

For the purpose of the analysis, four children (two from each ward) were paired together, with regard to the similarities between them. The data were then examined in relation to the amount and quality of the interaction between the children and other social actors, in particular the nurses. An attempt was then made to link this with the quality of care achieved in each ward setting.

There was more interaction between the nursing staff and the patients on the patient allocation ward than on the task allocation ward. The interaction was not exclusively related to the tasks that the nurses were performing. The nature of the interaction acknowledged the children as unique individuals, and there was more sociable interaction, which reinforced the individualised approach. The trained staff, including the sister in charge, did not exclude themselves from the interaction. The care was competent and compassionate.

The interaction on the task allocation ward usually focused around the tasks to be performed. It was of short duration and less frequent than that on the patient allocation ward. There was less interaction for sociable reasons. The style of the interaction appeared to be related to the task, rather than to the child as an individual. The trained staff engaged in less interaction with the children, and were, consequently, less visible in relation to the activities involving the delivery of direct patient care. The sister in charge was not observed interacting with either of the two children whose hospital experience was examined in detail. This tended to support the evidence provided by the admission and sister studies.

CONCLUSIONS

Discussion of the conclusions will focus on the crucial distinction between patient allocation as a system of work organisation and patient-centredness as a conceptual approach to nursing care. It will be essential to recognise that these two notions are different, as are those of task-centredness and task allocation. The data from the ward sister studies and the child studies firmly support these notions, which are central to the thesis. This began from the premise that there were assumed strengths and weaknesses associated with particular styles of work organisation, namely patient and task allocation, which could have profound implications on standards of patient care. In the process of examining these two notions, it was found that the orientation of the ward sister was crucial to what goes on in the ward – not only in terms of how the work is organised, but also for how the patient is perceived, the latter being of enormous importance to the standard of care that is ultimately delivered to the patient by the nursing staff.

Patient-/task-centredness is related to standards of care

In the absence of other definitions, standards of care have been defined in terms of patient-/task-centredness. The evidence from this study has been able to demonstrate the relationship between task-centredness and minimal standards of care.

This study has shown that patient- and task-centredness are likely to depend on how the ward sister conceptualises and practises her work rather than on how she organises the ward in terms of patient or task allocation. However, it seems more likely that a sister who is patient-centred will opt for a patient allocation style of work organisation, in the mistaken belief that this, of itself, will produce a more patient-centred approach by her staff. This does not preclude the possibility that other sisters may use a task allocation system of work organisation and, at the same time, be patient-centred in their conception of their work. This confirms the conclusion drawn by Boekholdt and Kanters (1978, p.323) that:

'team nursing provides only structural side conditions for face to face interaction between nurses and patients. Team nursing as a structural model is therefore not a sufficient condition for an increase in therapeutic behaviour.'

The evidence provided by the interviews and the ward sister study supports the view that the patient allocation sister saw her work in terms of the patients. This resulted in her nursing them as individuals, and, as a direct consequence of this, the quality of her interaction and the care that she personally delivered were of a high standard.

Conversely, the task allocation sister was task- rather than patient-orientated, the consequence of this being a lower quality of interaction and care on the part of the sister practitioner, who appeared to be dominated not only by tasks (which often did not directly affect standards of care one way or the other) but also by a particular hierarchy of tasks. Perhaps a significant message needs to be emphasised at this point, inasmuch as basic care is of vital importance to patients and must also be seen to be important to nurses, of whatever grade.

It became clear from the data that the sisters' behaviour was being reproduced by the rest of both the trained and the untrained staff (learners and auxiliaries). Therefore, the role models provided by the sisters in the setting of standards of care in relation to task- or patient-centredness appear to be vital.

Pembrey (1978) emphasised the importance of high role differentiation in order for sisters to be good managers. She did not, however, address the significance that the ward sister holds as a role model for the rest of the nursing staff. A major conclusion from this study has been that the ward sister must be seen to practise individualised nursing (rather than management) in order to be an effective role model for the delivery of such care. Of course, managing the nursing is crucial, but a very delicate balance needs to be maintained between managing the nursing and acting as a role model for the day-to-day interaction involved in the delivery of individualised patient care. Being a good manager and having medium/low role differentiation are perhaps not mutually exclusive, but appear to be essential components in the delivery of such care. From this present study, it would appear that it is not only the degree but also the nature of the sisters' role differentiation that is important. Stapleton (1983, p.22) emphasised this when she noted that:

> 'the crucial source of initiation to achieve patient care in a total sense must come from the ward sister.'

The maintenance and reproduction of task- and patient-centred systems

An analysis of the admission studies showed that there were considerable differences in the standards of care achieved on each of the two wards. However, the method of work organisation did not appear to provide an adequate explanation for the differences in these standards. All of the admitting nurses on each ward had had the same opportunity to achieve good quality interaction with the family unit. Why was it that the patient allocation nurses usually achieved this potential and the task allocation nurses invariably did not?

The admission procedure was allocated in the same way on each ward (as a task), but one of the striking differences between the two sets of admissions was the involvement of the trained staff on the patient allocation ward, where they were visibly interacting with the child and his/her family from the very beginning of their hospital experience. The trained staff sometimes actually admitted the child or, if not, were most likely to acknowledge him/her while admission was being completed. The trained staff also involved themselves in the subsequent care of the children. It is assumed that trained nurses are experts at nursing, and if they actually engage in nursing, this expertise will become more visible to those who are learning to nurse. It would seem, from the evidence in these data, that nursing is about being able to interact competently, compassionately and appropriately in three major arenas of care – technical, basic and psychosocial – for the duration of the patient's hospital stay.

In the task allocation ward, the trained staff were conspicuous by their absence from areas of direct nursing activity. The sister in charge was never observed interacting with children being admitted, despite, on several occasions, being in the immediate vicinity.

Broadley (1984), in an article in *Nursing Focus*, states:

'When a patient comes into a hospital he feels in danger of losing his identity, independence and his social and family status.'

This present study has concluded that this danger is minimised if the ward sister is prepared to set a good example in relation to maintaining the patient's self-identity, independence and social status; in other words, promoting a philosophy of individualised care, and, at the same time, acknowledging that patient-centred care implies negotiation between the patient and the nurses in relation to the form that the nursing care will take. The processes of negotiation and individual acknowledgement are initiated by the admission procedure, which is a ritual of some importance in establishing the therapeutic relationship between the hospital and the patient.

Patient-centredness means better total patient care

It became important to establish whether or not this notion of task- or patient-centredness, which had been found in the ward sisters' and the admission studies, was sustained during the subsequent care of the patients, and also whether or not it could be related to the standard of care that the patients received.

The evidence contained in the child studies tended to confirm the task-centredness of the task allocation ward nurses and the patient-centredness of the patient allocation ward nurses, with a corresponding association of minimum standards of care related to the former and high standards of care related to the latter.

It also became clear, from the data, that one of the assumptions made in the professional ideology was unsound – namely, that if patient allocation is practised, fewer nurses will be providing more nursing care to each patient. This present study has shown that similar numbers of nurses, in both the task allocation and patient allocation setting, interacted with the patient.

It could be said that one of the caveats of patient allocation and the individualistic approach is the assumption that all nurses are competent, caring and compassionate. It may be argued that if this is not so, the individual patient's burden of hospitalisation may be made more intolerable than it might have been in the task allocation situation, by the undiluted, individualistic attentions of an incompetent, uncaring or unfeeling nurse. However, it was found that the patient allocation children were not only cared for by their allocated nurses, but also by other members of the ward team. On the task allocation ward, although the work was allocated by task to specific nurses, the jobs were sometimes taken on by others in an ad hoc fashion. However, while the patient allocation nurses often combined being sociable with technical and basic work, as well as being sociable for its own sake, this did not appear to feature on the task allocation ward.

Webb (1981, p.373) expressed another fear in relation to an individualised approach when she stated:

> 'As a result of this breaking down of the barriers between nurses, patients and life outside, more of the patient is exposed to scrutiny and control. Areas which formerly did not enter into the treatment of the body have now become available for the treatment of the person. It is much more difficult for him to keep hidden these areas of life which are private and which he wants to keep to himself, for example, the quality of his marital relationship.'

The evidence in this study tends to dispel the anxiety as expressed by Webb (probably in relation to adult patients), in that invasion of privacy of all kinds was minimised. Taking into account that we invade the lives of children all the time, it is likely that this was facilitated by the fact that numerous nurses were involved in the patients' care, even in the patient allocation situation. Furthermore, an important prerequisite for the delivery of individualised care is the development, on the part of the nurse, of sensitivity to another's needs in relation to 'social space'.

In brief, the patient allocation nurses were patient-centred and did not confine the delivery of their care to their allocated patients.

The task allocation nurses did not confine themselves either to the job they were allocated or to the children who were batch-allocated to them. They tended to be task-centred. This would seem to suggest that a high quality of care is related to patient-centredness and a low quality of care to task-centredness. Since the nurses in both work situations did not confine themselves to the work remit laid down for them by the sister in the form of work lists or patient allocations (both sets of nurses worked across the board), the patient- or task-centredness must be to do with something other than the way in which the work is organised. This research has shown that, initially, it is to do with the role model provided by the sister in charge. The type of role model she provides (patient- or task-centred) is informed by the way in which she conceptualises her work: in terms of patients or tasks.

An Israeli study of role models (Dotan et al, 1986) emphasises this:

'One of the major implications derived from this study is that both teachers and head nurses must recognise that they are potential positive role models and so need to cultivate desirable affective and cognitive behaviour. This should be taken into consideration by their superiors in planning general and professional staff development and in preparing job descriptions.'

It would seem that it is this availability of the trained staff as role models for the actual delivery of nursing care (rather than concentrating exclusively on the organisation/administration of the ward) that is of crucial importance to the orientations of those who are learning to give the care. Of course, there were deviants in both settings, e.g. the patient allocation SEN who carried out a task-centred admission and the task allocation nurse who was patient-centred in her relationships with the children. The study by King et al (1971), into patterns of residential care, appeared to indicate that it was the type of training that carers received that dictated their work orientations. This current study would appear to challenge that assertion, since all the nurses had undergone a similar training experience, but, despite this, some of them were still patient-centred in the way that they carried out their work.

If the trained staff do not make themselves available as role models, then on whom are the learners to model themselves for the activity in which they are currently engaged i.e. nursing sick people? The General Nursing Council was aware of this problem and went so far as to state in 1983 (p.3) that:

'Care must be valued for its own sake and learners enabled to develop skills in maintaining prolonged relationships with patients and their relatives. New approaches to care are required in a variety of settings in co-operation with the family or other professional groups and voluntary organisations.'

It has been possible to conclude, thus far, that patient-centredness produces not only more psychosocial support, as evidenced in the admission studies, but also more basic care, as shown in the child studies. These are two important areas of care, much neglected in the past. Psychosocial needs are not often explicit and need high level skills to identify and meet them, whereas basic needs are often seen as requiring boring tasks to meet them and are left usually to the untrained staff to fulfil in a hierarchical setting.

Webb (1981, p.373) stated that:

'It could be argued that quality of care should be the sole criterion [for implementing the nurse process] but it has not yet been established whether this quality – however it may be defined and measured – is improved with a patient orientated mode.'

This study has attempted to begin a definition and measurement of quality of care. It has also demonstrated the beneficial effects of patient-centredness on the quality of care.

The emphasis of the study has shifted over time from initially seeking to establish whether there was any relationship between patterns of work organisation and quality of care, to recognising the significance of the ward sister as a role model for patient- or task-centredness. Although the nature of the contribution of the nursing process was not addressed, it would seem from the evidence so far that the nursing process would not of itself produce patient-centredness unless it was reinforced by the provision by the ward sister of the appropriate role model. The evolution of patient-centred care implies much social change. Moore (1968, p.366) succinctly outlines what this involves:

'Social change is the significant alteration of social structures (that is, patterns of social action and interaction), including consequences and manifestations of such structures embodied in norms (rules of conduct), values and cultural products and symbols.'

Additionally, it could be said that social change requires the motivation and goodwill of individual actors to support appropriate patterns of social action and interaction in order to effect the alteration. Are nurses equal to this enormous task? What strategies are required in order to facilitate the change?

RECOMMENDATIONS

The General Nursing Council (1983) has stated that:

'The need for patients and families to have adequate information, health education and their cultural and personal identity preserved must be recognised and their differing values accepted as part of their individuality which must not be ignored or destroyed.'

This research has shown that the development of patient-centred concepts on the part of the staff is crucial in order for this policy to become a reality. In the light of the research, it has been possible to make practical recommendations in the following areas.

Education for a more patient-centred approach

Perhaps one of the most fruitful ways forward, in order to achieve a universal patient-centred approach in nursing care, would be to alert trained nurses to the extent of the influence that they exert in the form of culture bearers and role models to those who are subordinate to them. This has significant implications for the development of continuing professional education, not only for clinical nurses, but also for tutorial staff, who should be prepared to demonstrate excellence and expertise in the practice of nursing. Hall (1977) refers to a study by Wilkinson (1973) which:

'throws light on the crucial role of the head nurse in acting as a "gate keeper" or "opinion leader" for the rest of her staff.' (p.48)

Pembrey (1978) described the sister as the 'key to nursing'. However, it would be unwise to confine the dissemination of this particular philosophy to the trained nurses already mentioned, because, as has previously been discussed, patient-centred care implies negotiation between the patient and the nurses in relation to the form that the care will take; this further implies knowledge sharing in order for the patient to make informed choices. This has profound implications for the delivery of all health care, inasmuch as it is likely that some patients will demand more discussion and adopt a more questioning approach to all issues of health care. In the light of this possible development, the education and training of all health personnel (including doctors) will need to be evaluated and modified.

Patient-centred policies

Dingwall and McIntosh (1978, p.164) note that:

> 'Both research into and debate on the quality of care have centred very largely on how excellence may be achieved, rather than why there are notable failures and how these may be prevented ... Rather than focusing exclusively on single events such as a surgical dressing or admission to hospital, is it not equally important to find what is actually going on in the everyday lives of patients and nurses?'

This present study has attempted to understand about both failure and excellence, by examining the everyday lives of patients and nurses; it has, nevertheless, been useful to examine the microcosm of a single event, in order to gain some sense of direction and confirmation of ideas in the analysis of the large scale scenario. In this instance, the single event was patient admission – as a result of abstracting this procedure from the data as a whole, it has been possible to suggest certain recommendations in relation to the approach to future admissions (see Brown forthcoming).

The role of the trained staff in all areas of patient care has been emphasised throughout this study. The involvement of the trained nurse in the admission procedure is crucial, not only in acting as role model but also in order to prevent feelings of social distance developing in staff–patient relationships, and to break down the notion of a task hierarchy. In order to reinforce the patient-centred approach, ward procedure manuals should include strategies for the psychosocial support of the patient, rather than just the instrumental aspects of admission that are emphasised at present (in a perfect world manuals would become redundant).

The point of admission is an important time for making the initial nursing assessment of the patient, as the first stage in the nursing process. This will be a pointless exercise if the nurse does not adopt a patient-centred approach; therefore, expert role models are essential in order to ensure that this is done effectively.

The role of the school of nursing in the development of patient-centredness

The Briggs Report (1972) asserted that learner nurses provide 75% of all bedside nursing care. (This is likely to continue for the foreseeable future, although changes in the status of the learner from apprentice to student are being implemented in some of the experimental training schemes set up by the English National Board.) It is, therefore, of considerable importance that learners be adequately prepared in the delivery of patient-centred care. The GNC (1983, p.1) acknowledge this when they state:

> 'The initial aim of nursing education is to provide for the learner an appropriate balance between theory and practice, so that newly qualified nurses have the knowledge, skills and attitudes necessary to enable them to provide systematic individual patient/client-centred care.'

Both ward sisters and nurse tutors must work together to achieve the integration of theory with practice, and appropriate teaching tools should be developed to facilitate this.

The physical resources available for the use of the children and their families in this study were sometimes rather stretched. However, the hospital staff, by using a little flexibility and ingenuity, could utilise existing facilities more effectively for the benefit of the family unit. One has sometimes been left with the impression that hospitals in general, and wards in particular, are organised the way they are for the benefit of the staff, rather than for those with the greatest needs i.e. the patients. The research has shown that, judging from the outside, patients have a better experience of hospital if a patient-centred approach is adopted. The overwhelming message is, therefore, to urge the nursing profession to develop more patient-centredness and to be quite clear what this entails. This section on recommendations began with a quote from the GNC, but nurses must be alert to the fact that official policy can be unsound and misguided. The nursing profession is currently experiencing considerable pressure from the statutory body (UKCC) to move towards a patient allocation with a nursing process system of work organisation. This present research (along with that of Metcalfe, 1982) has shown that it is likely that the nature of the work organisation is immaterial to the patient- or task-centredness of the nursing staff. It cannot be said too often that it is important to discriminate between patient allocation as a system of work organisation and patient-centredness as a conceptual approach to nursing. These two things are not the same; they are different, as are task-centredness and task allocation. The emphasis for change needs to be shifted from the work organisation to the support and development of the ward sister, in order to help her to focus on the patient in her work conceptualisation. A fundamental assumption that has been made throughout this argument is that the function of ward sisters is related to nursing patients rather than to concentrating completely on the management of the ward. This opens up a whole range of questions outside the remit of this research, not least of which is, if we are not training nurses to nurse patients, what are we training them for? Perhaps we should not expect one individual to have to be all things to all people.

FURTHER RESEARCH

This research has generated more questions than it has answered. It has not been possible to address several areas of major importance to the development of patient-centred care. These are discussed below in relation to the various categories used as a framework for this final chapter.

What makes a trained nurse task- or patient-centred?

One of the major issues generated by the ward sister study is 'What makes nurses think of their work in terms of patients or tasks?' Replication of this part of the study would probably show that there are degrees of patient- and task-centredness – and the reasons for the particular orientation are likely to be multifactorial and extremely complex. However, this present research has suggested that a possible fruitful line of enquiry could be the influence of previous role models and significant others to the trained nurse's present orientation towards her work. Pembrey (1978) has also suggested that ward sisters who are generally and professionally well educated tend to manage the ward in terms of individual patients.

Replication of the ward sister study is also essential to check out the characteristics of patient- and task-centredness that have been identified in the two ward sisters.

The study was in depth and detailed, which was extremely important in order to establish the parameters of an area of nursing that has been under-researched in the past. By doing this small scale, in-depth study, the way has been paved for further work by defining the 'nature of the beast'.

Patient satisfaction in patient-centred admissions

It would also have been useful to have measured the level of satisfaction experienced by the patients and their families as a result of the two different orientations, particularly since even the admissions that were patient-centred could in no sense be described as perfect.

The effects of patient- and task-centredness in relation to patients and nurses

Two important areas of investigation suggested by this study focus on the effects of patient- and task-centredness in relation to (a) the patients and (b) the nurses. Although this current study has asserted that the patient experiences a better quality of care, this quality has tended to defer to professional definitions of standards. A closer examination of how the patient perceives a task- or patient-centred approach may reveal that these perceptions may not conform to those defined by the nurse researcher, or, if there is some agreement, that the different components of what constitutes quality of care may be prioritised differently by the patient.

In relation to the nurses, Menzies (1970) has suggested that task allocation is a means by which nurses fragment the patient into a series of tasks, and thereby avoid the necessity to engage emotionally with the patient. This study suggests that it is the way in which the patient is perceived, rather than the actual work organisation, that influences the degree of emotional involvement between the nursing staff and the patients. The different levels of stress that may be associated with patient- and task-centredness have not been addressed, and this is clearly very important. Much concern is currently being expressed about who cares for the carers, and an examination of this issue would be helpful in informing those who support the nurse in her clinical work.

Towards the theory and practice of individualised care

The contribution of theoretical models in nursing to the understanding of patient care was not within the remit of this research. However, in view of the current major debates and anxieties in relation to nursing theory, it would be remiss of this researcher not to discuss tentative relationships between this research and these contemporary developments.

Hardy (1982) notes:

'In an examination of some models it was discovered that narrow interpretations of nursing by the nurse theorists has created specific difficulties in the presentation of what nursing is and what affects it.'

She goes on to criticise the failure of most nursing theorists to address the characteristics of nurses as individuals and how these contribute to nursing. She acknowledges the early efforts of Abdellah et al (1960) to bear this in mind:

'While they cultivated a primary idea which centred on the client, the nurse herself was to be considered also. Germination did not occur as the up and coming nurse theorist gardeners chose to nurture the main area of Abdellah's treatise, that is, patient centred care.'

Hardy (1982) applauds the ideas of Robert Chin, who suggested that the nurse (change agent) should create her own system. Chin (1974) states that:

'Helpers of change are prone at times not to see that their own systems as change agents have boundaries, tensions, stresses and strains, equilibria and feedback mechanisms which may be just as much part of the problem as are similar aspects of the "client systems".'

Nurse theorists have, in the main, addressed the nature of the patient and the care setting, the nature of health/illness and nursing itself, and, while Hardy (1982) implies approval of what she sees as a shift from the medical (disease-oriented) model of care to an emphasis on patients, she believes that 'one track is one track, however defined'.

This current research has endeavoured not to be one track. It has tried to focus on nurses as well as on patients, and has entertained the idea of adding a fifth parameter to nursing theory – i.e. the nature of the nurse – as this would appear to be paramount in achieving what seems to be an exceedingly attractive goal, that of patient-centred care.

References

Abdellah F G, Beland I L, Martin A and Matheney R V (1960) *Patient-Centred Approaches to Nursing.* New York: Macmillan.

Adelman C, Jenkins D and Kemmis S (1975) Re-thinking case study: Notes from the Second Cambridge Conference. *Cambridge Journal of Education,* **6**: 139–150.

Auld M (1968) Team nursing in a maternity hospital. *Midwife and Health Visitor,* **4**: 242–245.

Bendall E (1975) *So You Passed, Nurse?* London: Royal College of Nursing.

Bernstein B (1975) *Class, Codes and Control,* Vol. 3: *Towards Theory of Educational Transmissions.* London: Routledge and Kegan Paul.

Boekholdt M E and Kanters H W (1978) Team nursing in a general hospital – theory, results and limitations. *Journal of Occupational Psychology,* **5**: 315–325.

Bowlby J (1951) *Maternal Care and Mental Health,* 2nd edn. Geneva: World Health Organisation.

Briggs Report (1972) *Report of the Committee on Nursing.* London: HMSO.

Broadley K (1984) Stress and insomnia. *Nursing Focus,* **5**(5):11.

Brown G W (1973) The mental hospital as an institution. *Social Science of Medicine,* **7**: 407–424. Oxford: Pergamon Press.

Brown R A (1986) *The Social Organisation of Work in Two Paediatric Wards in Relation to Patient and Task Allocation.* MPhil thesis, University of Warwick.

Burgess R G (ed.) (1982) *Field Research: A Sourcebook and Field Manual.* London: George Allen and Unwin.

Chavasse J (1976) *Patient Allocation Compared to Task Allocation.* Unpublished conference paper. RCN Research Conference, Edinburgh.

Chavasse J (1981) From task assignment to patient allocation. A change evaluation. *Journal of Advanced Nursing,* **6**: 137–145.

Chin R (1974) The utility of systems models and developmental models for practitioners. In: *Conceptual Models for Nursing Practice.* eds. Riehl J P and Roy C. New York: Appleton–Century–Crofts.

Clamp C G L (1984) *Learning Through Incidents.* Unpublished MPhil thesis, University of London.

Cleary J (1977) Distribution of nursing attention in a children's ward. *Nursing Times* Occasional Paper, **73**(28):93–96.

Cleary J (1979) Demands and responses. The effects of the style of work allocation on the distribution of nursing attention. In: *Beyond separation*, eds. Hall D and Stacey M. London: Routledge and Kegan Paul.

Consumers' Association (1980) *Children in hospital*. A *Which?* Campaign Report. London: Consumers' Association.

Consumers' Association (1985) Children in Hospital. *Which?* magazine, pp. 184–185.

Corwin G (1965) The professional employee: a study of conflict in nursing roles. In: *Social Interaction and Patient Care*, eds. Skipper J K and Leonard R C. New York : Lippincott.

Coser R L (1963) Alienation and the social structure. In: *The Hospital in Modern Society*, pp. 231–265. ed. Freidson E. London: Free Press.

De la Cuesta C (1983) The nursing process: from development to implementation. *Journal of Advanced Nursing*, **8**: 365–371.

Denzin N K (1970) *The Research Act in Sociology*. London: Butterworth.

Dingwall R and McIntosh J (eds.) (1978) *Readings in the Sociology of Nursing*. London: Churchill Livingstone.

Dickoff J, James P and Semradek J (1975) 8–4 Research, Part 1: A stance for nursing research. *Nursing Research*, **24**(2):89 Part 2: Designing nursing research – eight points of encounter. *Nursing Research*, **24**(3).

Dotan M, Krulik T, Bergman R, Eckerling S and Schatzman M (1986) Role models in nursing. *Nursing Times* Occasional Paper, **82**(3): 55–57.

Douglas J D (1976) *The Relevance of Sociology*. New York: Appleton–Century–Crofts.

Evers H K (1984) *Patients' Experiences and Social Relations in Geriatric Wards*. Unpublished PhD thesis, University of Warwick.

Foreman P B (1971) Execution of the research design: case studies. In: *Research Methods: Issues and Insights*, eds. Franklin B J and Osborne H W. London: Wadsworth.

Fox D (1966) *Fundamentals of Research in Nursing*. New York: Appleton–Century–Crofts.

Franklin B J and Osborne H W (1971) *Research Methods: Issues and Insights*. London: Wadsworth.

Fretwell J E (1978) *Teaching and Learning in the Ward Situation*. Unpublished PhD thesis, University of Warwick.

Fretwell J E (1980) An inquiry into the ward learning environment. *Nursing Times* Occasional Paper, **76**(16): 69–75.

General Nursing Council (1983) Educational Policy, June 83/13/A.

Gold R L (1971) Roles in sociological observations. In: *Research Methods: Issues and Insights*, Franklin B J and Osborne H W. London: Wadsworth.

Grant N (1979) *Time to Care*. London: Royal College of Nursing.

Hall D J (1975) *Social Relations and Innovations: Play in Children's Wards*. Unpublished PhD thesis, University College of Swansea.

Hall D J (1977) *Social Relations and Innovation*. London: Routledge and Kegan Paul.

Hall D J and Stacey M (eds) (1979) *Beyond Separation*. London: Routledge and Kegan Paul.

Haralambos M (1980) *Sociology Themes and Perspectives*. Slough: University Tutorial Press.

Hardy L K (1982) Nursing models and research – a restricting view?

Journal of Advanced Nursing, **7**: 447–451.

Hawthorn P J (1974) *Nurse I want my Mummy*. London: Royal College of Nursing.

Holt K S and Reynell J L (1970) *Observations of Children*. London: National Association of Mental Health.

Hunt J M and Marks-Maran D J (1980) *Nursing Care Plans*. London: HM & M.

Jacobs R (1979) The meaning of hospital: denial of emotions. In: *Beyond Separation*. eds. Hall D J and Stacey M. London: Routledge and Kegan Paul.

Jenkinson V M (1958) Group or team nursing. *Nursing Times*, **54**(3):62–64; **54**(4): 92–93.

Jenkinson V M (1961) Team nursing. *Nursing Times*. **57**(9):264–266.

Johnson M M and Martins H W (1965) A sociological analysis of the nurse role. In: *Social Interaction and Patient Care*, eds. Skipper J K and Leonard R C. Philadelphia: Lippincott.

Jolly J (1981) *Communicating with Children in Hospital*. London: HM&M.

King R D, Raynes N V and Tizard J (1971) *Patterns in Residential Care*. London: Routledge and Kegan Paul.

Kratz C R (1974) *Problems in the Care of the Long-term Sick in the Community*. Unpublished PhD thesis, University of Manchester.

Lazarsfeld P F and Barton A (1971) Qualitative measurement in the social sciences. In: *Research Methods: Issues and Insights*, Franklin B J and Osborne H W. London: Wadsworth.

Lelean S (1973) *Ready for Report Nurse?* London: Royal College of Nursing.

Lelean S (1980) Research in nursing. *Nursing Times* Occasional Paper, **76**(3): 5–8.

Luker K A (1980) *Health Visiting and the Elderly: An Experimental Study to Evaluate the Effects of Focused Health Visitor Intervention on Elderly Women Living Alone at Home*. Unpublished PhD thesis, University of Edinburgh.

Lundberg G A (1971) Alleged obstacles to social science. In: *Research Methods: Issues and Insights*, Franklin B J and Osborn H W. London: Wadsworth.

Marks-Maran D (1978) Patient allocation versus task allocation in relation to the nursing process. *Nursing Times*, **74**(10): 413–416.

Matthews A (1972) Total patient care in the ward. *Nursing Mirror*, 11 April, pp.29–31.

Menzies I E P (1970) *The Functioning of Social Systems as a Defence Against Anxiety*. London: Tavistock Institute of Human Relations.

Menzies I E P (1975) *The Psychological Welfare of Young Children Making Long Stays in Hospital*. London: Tavistock Institute of Human Relations.

Metcalfe C A (1982) *A Study of a Change in the Method of Organising the Delivery of Nursing Care in a Ward of a Maternity Hospital*. Unpublished PhD thesis, University of Manchester.

Mitchell A (1984) The nursing process debate. *Nursing Times*, **80**(19): 28–32.

Moore W E (1968) *Social Change. International Encyclopaedia of the Social*

Sciences, Vol. 14. London: Collier MacMillan.

Pembrey S M (1975) From work routines to patient allocation. *Nursing Times*, **31**(45): 1768–1772.

Pembrey,, S.M. (1978) *The Role of the Ward Sister in the Management* of *Nursing. A Study of the Organisation of Nursing on an Individualised Patient Basis*. Unpublished PhD thesis, University of Edinburgh.

Pembrey S M (1980) *The Ward Sister – Key to Nursing*. London: Royal College of Nursing.

Pembrey S M (1983) Can clinical nursing be managed? *Nursing Mirror*, **157**(21): 26–27.

Perry E L (1968) *Ward Administration and Teaching. The Work of the Ward Sister*. London: Baillière Tindall.

Pill R (1970) The sociological aspects of the case-study sample. In: *Hospitals, Children and their Families*, Stacey M, Deardon R, Pill R and Robinson D. London: Routledge and Kegan Paul.

Platt Report (1959) *Welfare of Children in Hospital*. Report of the Committee, Ministry of Health. London: HMSO

Plumpton M (1978) Experiments in nurse/patient allocation. *Nursing Times*, **74**(10): 417–419.

Revans R W (1964) *Standards for Morale: Cause and Effect in Hospitals*. Nuffield Provincial Hospitals Trust. Oxford: Oxford University Press.

Robertson J (1958) *Young Children in Hospital*, 1st edn. London: Tavistock.

Royal College of Nursing (1956) *Observations and Objections: A Statement of Nursing Policy*. London: Royal College of Nursing.

Royal College of Nursing (1980) *Standards of Nursing Care*. Discussion document. London: Royal College of Nursing.

Scales M (1958) *Handbook For Ward Sisters*. London: Baillière Tindall and Cox.

Schatzman L and Strauss A L (1973) *Field Research*. Englewood Cliffs, NJ: Prentice Hall.

Spencer J (1983) Research with a human touch. *Nursing Times*, **79**(12): 24–27.

Stacey M (1969) *Methods of Social Research*. Oxford: Pergamon Press.

Stacey M, Deardon R, Pill R and Robinson D (1970) *Hospitals, Children and their Families*. London: Routledge and Kegan Paul.

Stapleton M F (1983) *Ward Sisters – Another Perspective*. London: Royal College of Nursing.

Wainwright P and Burnip S (1983) QUALPACS at Burford. *Nursing Times*, **79**(5): 36–38; **79**(33): 26–27.

Walker V H (1967) *Nursing and Ritualistic Practice*. New York: Macmillan.

Wandelt M and Ager J (1974) *Quality Patient Care Scale*. New York: Appleton–Century–Crofts.

Wax R H (1971) *Doing Fieldwork: Warnings and Advice*. Chicago: University of Chicago Press.

Webb C (1981) Classification and framing: a sociological analysis of task-centred nursing and the nursing process. *Journal of Advanced Nursing*, **6**: 369–376.

Wilkinson G S (1973) Interaction patterns and staff response to psychiatric innovations. *Journal of Health and Social Behaviour,* **14**: 323–329.

Wright H F (1960) Observational child study. In: *Handbook of Research Methods in Child Development,* ed. Musson P H. New York: Wiley.

Yin R K (1984) *Case Study Research Design and Methods. Applied Social Research Methods,* Vol. 5, Beverley Hills: Sage Publications.